OXFORD MEDICAL PUBLICATIONS

The mouth, the face, and the mind

The mouth, the face, and the mind

Edited by

CHARLOTTE FEINMANN

Reader and
Honorary Consultant Liaison Psychiatrist
Eastman Dental Institute and Hospital, London
and
Royal Free and University College Medical School, London

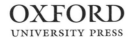

OXFORD
UNIVERSITY PRESS

OXFORD
UNIVERSITY PRESS

Great Clarendon Street, Oxford OX2 6DP

Oxford University Press is a department of the University of Oxford.
It furthers the University's objectives of excellence in research, scholarship,
and education by publishing worldwide in

Oxford New York

Athens Auckland Bangkok Bogotá Buenos Aires Calcutta
Cape Town Chennai Dar es Salaam Delhi Florence Hong Kong Istanbul
Karachi Kuala Lumpur Madrid Melbourne Mexico City Mumbai
Nairobi Paris São Paulo Singapore Taipei Tokyo Toronto Warsaw
and associated companies in Berlin Ibadan

Oxford is a registered trade mark of Oxford University Press
in the UK and in certain other countries

Published in the United States
by Oxford University Press, Inc., New York

A catalogue record for this book is available from the British Library

Library of Congress Cataloging in Publication Data
(Data available)

ISBN 0 19 263062 8

Typset by Downdell, Oxford
Printed in Great Britain
on acid-free paper by
Biddles Ltd
Guildford and King's Lynn

Foreword

This book, with its emphasis on the head and on pain, is full of challenge and intriguing ideas. As soon as we animals began to move in one preferred direction, there were huge consequences. The major sense organs all migrated to the prow as did the tools for eating, expression, and aggression. We are not even the extreme in this respect. The mouse has placed whisking whiskers on its nose which are in effect exploring fingers and which are supplied by the infraorbital nerve (by far the largest nerve in a mouse, and three times the size of the sciatic nerve). Only we advanced monkeys have slightly reversed this trend by standing on our two feet to liberate our hands to take over some of the face functions of other animals and to use hands to explore, feed, and fight. As the source of information and of action migrated to the head so did the neural machinery. Sir Charles Bell did us little favour by labelling the trigeminal nerve as the spinal nerve of the head as though the face represented just another of the body's segments. It is true that the fifth nerve has the same general plan with its vast Gasserian ganglion as the equivalent of the dorsal root ganglia and its motor component as the ventral roots. This crucial early nineteenth century observation really set the scene for academic medicine and dentistry and the leit motif for this book. Cell by cell I know of no fundamental difference between individual cells of the head and those of the rest of the body. Therefore, following the present day popular reductionist approach, one might predict that there are no fundamental differences in the function or malfunction of tissues in the face or in the rest of the body. That would seem a reasonable approach if one were dealing with malfunctions of small groups of cells as in inflammation or carcinoma. The question set by Dr Feinmann and her colleagues is whether pain in the face and mouth is simply another example of the pains encountered elsewhere in the body and should be analysed and treated as such.

The clinical description of oral-facial pains in this book makes fascinating reading for anyone. There are clear examples of disorders apparently unique to the head. The most obvious is trigeminal neuralgia which is specific both in its symptomatology and treatment. Certainly there is no such dramatic disorder apparent elsewhere. Does its existence mean that there is some particular fragility in the trigeminal system? There are, of course, painful tender spots which appear elsewhere in the body but they differ from the specific trigger points of trigeminal neuralgia which are fired by superficial moving stimuli, frequently respond to antiepileptics and to neurosurgery directed at the fifth nerve. Yet there is a common puzzle in these two conditions. No pathology has been located either in the trigger points or along the course of the peripheral nerve. Could it be that sensory systems can drift into highly localized hyperexcitable states? Other examples of apparently unique complaints are the various headaches for which there seems no equivalent elsewhere. But is that true on more careful thought? The common tension headache has the pain localized in the head but is clearly a widespread disorder with many systemic signs and symptoms. Migraine pain is limited to the head but changes so many other parts of the body that it is now considered more an encephalopathy. The headaches like trigeminal neuralgia lack an observed pathology and are pain states without an appropriate localized peripheral cause. The muscle tension of tension headaches is not adequate to provoke the pain and the vascular changes of vascular (migraine) headaches do not explain the pain. The specificity of head pains may on occasions be an artefact of the way in which they are defined. For example, the temporo-mandibular joint syndrome is by definition related to the temporo-mandibular joint. The anatomical label does not differentiate it from other idiopathic disorders in neck, shoulders, arms, or back. We must all face a crisis in understanding pain when the number of idiopathic disorders and patients with these disorders far out-number those with an appropriate pain whose cause is defined by some overt pathology. A patient with a toothache and an infected cavity triggers an explanation and a therapy. We are so enchanted by the rationality of that successful process that we are driven to search for the 'cavity' in anyone complaining of pain. I fully agree with this approach since it could be that the 'cause' of a pain is hidden from us by our crude and inefficient ways of diagnosing disorders particularly of soft tissue and by our complete inability to detect subtle disorders of conduction pathways both in the peripheral and central nervous system. The search for these causes must continue but the problem has been made more difficult by the recent science of pain mechanisms which show a plastic reactive system where a frank disorder in the periphery can migrate to trigger abnormalities in the peripheral nerves and then proceed into the central cells of the medulla and further into the brain stem. The classical approach to pain is a bottom-up route which sees the origin in the periphery of pain producing nerve impulses. This approach has severe practical difficulties.

This book takes an alternate line with huge skill. It is in no way contradictory to the classical one but is complementary. It begins not with a nerve impulse but with what the patient in pain does and says. No-one can feel pain or anything else unless they pay attention. The dramatic examples on battle fields and sports fields of people with obvious injuries but no pain are caused by attention being locked on some other target. Distraction is the commonest folk medicine for pain and it works. Anxiety locks the attention and amplifies its target. When attention is captured, the whole body changes and muscles contract to inspect the source of pain and to guard it and to lock the zone into immobility. Relaxation is a treatment for pain. Pains are never pure pains. They come in a package with misery, fear, and worry. As pains persist, depression is added to emphasize the anxiety.

We are in a very exciting phase of science where brain images are being made of people in pain. They give no support at all to the serial picture of Descartes that sensation precedes emotion and that both have their special locations in the brain. These qualities seem simultaneously created which lends support to those cognitive therapies which explain meanings. The most surprising outcome of these pain studies has been the failure to identify separate sensory areas divorced from areas associated with movement. Pain may well be an awareness of a motor plan which aims to cure the pain. Pain is then a need state like hunger and thirst. When a patient believes that an action has been taken to relieve the state, there is a response called the placebo reaction. The question 'Is this pain real or mental?' has no meaning.

The very honest approach in this book moves beyond that crude misunderstanding and shows how to intrude on the patients' misery with open-hearted honesty. It does not require the patient to fit some theory of causation before they are given the honour of skilled help.

Patrick D. Wall
Professor of Physiology

This book is dedicated to Jessie, Charlie, and John,
with thanks for their patience and help.

Contents

Contributors

Dr Susan J. Cunningham   Lecturer in Orthodontics, Eastman Dental Institute

Dr Charlotte Feinmann   Reader and Honorary Consultant Liaison Psychiatrist, Eastman Dental Institute and Hospital, Royal Free and University College Medical School

Dr Lesley Glover   Chartered Clinical Psychologist, Sub-department of Clinical Health Psychology, University College London

Dr Sheelah Harrison   Specialist Registrar, Maxillo-facial Surgery, Eastman Dental Hospital and University College Hospital

Dr Richard Ibbetson   Dean for External Affairs, Eastman Dental Hospital

Ms Stephanie Jones   Chartered Clinical Health Psychologist, Chronic Fatigue Service, St Bartholomew's Hospital

Mr Geir Madland   MRC Research Fellow, Department of Psychiatry and Behavioural Science, Royal Free and University College Medical School

Acknowledgement

I would like to thank all the patients and colleagues from whom I have learnt and those colleagues who have supported me. There are too many to mention individually. I thank Jenny McGillion for typing the manuscript.

Introduction

Chronic orofacial symptoms affect the mouth and face; symptoms include pain, disturbances in jaw movement, sensation, salivation, or ulceration. These symptoms are often revealed to be due to emotional disturbance, and appropriate medical treatment of such problems benefits both patients and the health services. The association of emotional and mental suffering with the mouth may be interpreted in a number of ways, based on the anatomical, physiological, and developmental aspects of oral function. Not only do the lips, tongue, and oral mucosa have an exceptionally rich sensory innervation, but also the muscles of emotional expression gain their principal insertions around the mouth. Furthermore, the cortical projection of this part of the peripheral nervous system is large compared to, say, the trunk.

In infancy, the mouth plays a vital role in exploration, feeding, and establishing the affectional bonds with the mother. This process has been studied by ethologists, psychoanalysts, and psychologists. All agree from widely differing points of view on the mouth's fundamental importance in this formative period and in later life.

Freud postulated that not only do the experiences and management of the oral stage of development determine important personality traits, but that problems at this stage lead to a predisposition to certain kinds of depression in later life. On the other hand, the learning theorists see the role of the mouth as providing a highly specialized and delicate field, which may acquire at critical periods in the course of growth, such as childhood, adolescence, and adult life, a special capacity for the experience of pleasurable function or emotional pain. Certainly, all agree that tasting and eating, speaking, kissing, and other forms of sexual contact give the oral region a special significance in every patient's thinking and feeling.

This, of course, creates a latent complex situation for dental surgeons, making treatment of the mouth and teeth difficult. Not only have they to prevent or control anticipated pain but they may also be interfering with other aspects of the emotional well-being of their patients. Dentists must therefore be able to recognize the orofacial manifestations of psychiatric disorders, which in certain instances they may unwittingly trigger off or localize themselves.

It is important at the outset to understand that these orofacial problems are not a figment of the patient's imagination. The emotions can disturb a wide variety of hormonal, vascular, and muscular functions, all of which may produce peripheral changes varying from pain, dysfunction, and xerostomia to ulceration.

In some situations the casual relationship may be evident, as for instance, in postpuerperal or menopausal depression, where alterations in sex hormones and amine metabolism may precipitate an emotional disturbance, usually called an affective disorder, and also produce peripheral symptoms such as a burning tongue, facial pain, and pruritus. In other cases the neurophysiological mechanism is not apparent.

CLINICAL CONSIDERATIONS

The many different orofacial disorders include tension headache, neckache, facial arthromyalgia (temporomandibular joint dysfunction), atypical facial pain, atypical odontalgia, and oral dysaesthesia. Other disorders such as 'phantom bite', factitious ulceration, or an obsessional preoccupation with some part of the face (body dysmorphic disorder, BDD), may represent a more serious psychological disturbance.

Unfortunately, these disorders tend to be separated by their clinical presentation, so that patients with oral, joint, and muscle pain are seen and treated by dental specialists and the rest by neurologists, otolaryngologists, or psychiatrists, with little genuine collaboration between the specialities. Central to the understanding of these problems is that patients who are emotionally disturbed frequently present with physical symptoms, and that recognition of such an emotional disturbance benefits both the individual and the health service (Bridges and Goldberg 1988). However, recognition and appropriate treatment can only occur when a common understanding and classification of these disorders are reached.

Chronic idiopathic facial pain is a common problem, up to 10 per cent of the population are affected at some time in life (Von Knorff 1998). The main focus of this text is concerned with the recognition and management of such pain and reflects the clinical and research experience of the authors. Other subjects covered are the management of anxiety and psychological aspects of head and neck surgery.

REFERENCES

Bridges, K. and Goldberg, D. P. (1988) Somatic presentations of psychiatric illness in primary care settings. *Journal of Psychosomatic Research*, **32**, 137–44.
Von Knorff, M. (1998) Health Service Research and Temporomandibular Pain. In: *Progress in Research and Management*, vol. 4. pp. 227. IASP Press, Seattle. Ed. Sesole, B., Bryant, B. and Dionne, R. A.

1

The presentation of emotional disturbance and psychiatric illness to the dentist: recognition and definition

Charlotte Feinmann

INTRODUCTION

Dentists are used to seeing patients with straightforward problems, which respond to appropriate treatment and do not recur. Patients presenting to both medical and dental practitioners are, however, more likely to complain solely of physical symptoms than emotional disturbance, which may only become apparent when the patient is examined by a psychiatrist. Persistent somatic complaints may then lead to specialist referral. Frequently, the specialists consulted have neither the time nor the training required to recognize and discuss emotional problems, and a number of investigations are carried out before a diagnosis, or more often non-diagnosis, of organic disease is made. The investigation and management of such patients utilizes an inordinate amount of dental and medical practitioners' time and energy. Not only do negative investigations cost money, they may also demoralize both patient and practitioner. What is required is some means of identifying emotional disturbance and therefore restricting the number of physical investigations. The term 'somatization' is used to describe symptoms misattributed by patients to physical disease.

IDENTIFICATION OF EMOTIONAL DISTURBANCE

The aims of this chapter are to describe the diagnostic categories currently available for classifying patients with chronic pain or some other somatic problem, and to attempt to clarify the contribution psychiatry can make in the assessment of these patients.

Many people are under stress and unhappy but do not seek help. A number of selection processes happen before an individual becomes a patient. From a large number of potential patients, an unknown proportion elect to become, or are selected to become, actual patients. Becoming a patient is the end result of a complex chain of events that depend upon the nature of the symptomatology, alternative forms of treatment, availability of treatment facilities, economic factors, and a willingness to accept a patient's role.

A further complicating fact is that many of the patients who consult a GP, dentist, or hospital specialist with problems that are psychiatric in origin, frequently go unrecognized (Shepherd *et al.* 1966; Goldberg and Blackwell 1970). When examined by a psychiatrist, 25–70 per cent of hospital and general practice patients are reported to show previously unrecognized psychiatric disturbance.

The failure to recognize psychiatric problems may be due to the fact that patients may focus on somatic complaints and deny affective complaints (Katon 1982). Kroneke and Mangelsdorff (1989) examined the records of 1000 out-patients investigated over a 3-year period and found that only 16 per cent of patients had an organic cause for their symptoms. The cost of discarding an organic diagnosis was particularly high for certain symptoms, such as headache (US$7778). Out-patients in primary care who have mental disorders utilize more health resources, have greater disability, and more medical hospitalization (Katon and Gonzales 1994). Early recognition of psychological factors may prevent unnecessary investigations and costly interventions, including further consultations with other hospital specialists (Katon *et al.* 1990). Co-morbid psychiatric and psychological disorders have also been shown to contribute to long hospital stays (Soroway *et al.* 1995).

It is possible that a similar proportion of patients with minor psychiatric disorders present to dental as to medical practitioners, but dentists receive even less training than their medical counterparts to aid recognition and management of such disorders (Blinkhorn *et al.* 1979). The rest of this chapter will detail the recognition and assessment of patients with emotional problems who present to dental practitioners. When Cooper (1980) asked practising dentists to list their sources of stress, coping with difficult patients was the most important. It seems that if patients could be helped, dentists would also benefit.

BECOMING A PATIENT

What makes a patient seek help at a particular point in time? Patients may present with dental problems because they are under stress and a previously tolerable discomfort becomes unbearable. The association of stress and illness is complicated. It is known that life events and psychiatric illness are associated with suppression of the immune response and that a disease process as apparently simple as a bacterial throat infection, is influenced by personality factors. Meyer and Haggerty (1962) showed that in young children there was no relationship between episodes of streptococcal illness and the number or type of streptococci present, but a close relationship with the incidence of family crisis in those children.

ILLNESS BEHAVIOUR

This term was introduced by Pilowsky (1969) to describe the persistence of an inappropriate way of perceiving, evaluating, and acting in relation to health symptoms. Although these behaviours are defined multi-factorially, they are understood largely as the desire to elicit increased care from others. Shepherd (1995) has studied the illness behaviour of people injured in violence and has argued that doctors should be more proactive to improve the protection and support of vulnerable people involved in violence and to deal with psychological sequelae of violence.

Antecedents of illness

Life events

The first step (Fig. 1.1) is the influence of an unpleasant event. During the past four decades there has been considerable emphasis on the association of stress and disease. Early work examined the effect of loss on feelings of helplessness, later the concept of stress as a consequence of change in life developed.

A wide variety of events occur in a person's life which elicit responses. These life events may be positive (getting married, promotion, having a baby) or negative (bereavements, marital break-up), and the degree to which an individual responds to any one type of event is highly dependent upon the personal characteristics of that individual. Coping mechanisms and the presence or absence of social support may significantly modify the degree of stress to the individual. Environmental variables may also shape emotional response, so that danger events are followed by anxious symptoms, and loss by depressive symptoms.

A wide variety of ill health has been associated with increased life change. These include such diverse disorders as depression, myocardial infarction, appendicitis, and facial pain. It would, however, be a gross oversimplification to view stress as the only important variable in the elaboration of patterns of illness. Ford (1983) suggests the following ways in which stress may modify the disease process (see Fig. 1.1).

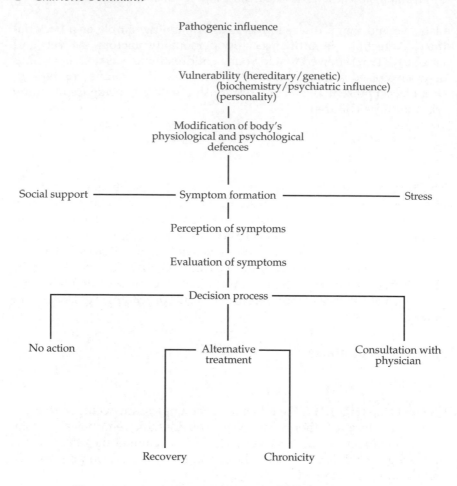

Fig. 1.1 A schematic view of the process of illness and disease.

1.   Stress, either physical or psychological, may modify the body's defences; for example, immune function has been shown to be reduced in high-stress situations. A large literature, under the general heading of psychoneuroimmunology, has developed (Ader 1981; Kiecolt-Glaser and Glaser 1992). The majority of studies have documented the downward modulation of immune system function as a result of stress or adverse life events, and there is evidence of upward regulation of immune system function as a result of psychological intervention. This may account for the increase in both minor and major illness in the bereaved.

2.   Stress may induce emotional responses that lead to physiological change, such as increased muscle tension or arterial spasm accounting

for facial pain, headache, backache, migraine, spastic colon, and a variety of psychosomatic symptoms (Holmes and Wolffe 1952), although there is little support in the literature for muscle contraction as a major cause of pain (Feinmann 1988).

3. Stress may intensify or alter the perception of concurrently existing physical symptoms (Mechanic 1972), so that a previously bearable tooth-ache becomes intolerable and emergency help is necessary. Amplification of normal bodily sensations may lead to somatization (conviction of physical ill health) or hypochondriasis (fear of physical illness).

4. Stress may also influence a decision to seek medical help (Tessler *et al*. 1976). An episode of acute stress with coincident dental treatment may lead to long-term pain, for which the dentist is blamed (Kent 1984).

5. Stress may induce the acceptance of the sick and invalid role and therefore reduce external stress (Mechanic 1972). This may account for 'surgeon shopping' or 'doctor hopping' shown by those constantly seeking reassurance. This search for help becomes self-defeating if the patient is passed from specialist to specialist.

Personality

Personality affects not only the way in which patients respond to and report symptoms but also the selection processes that determine the level of care at which treatment is received. There is significant variation in the way people perceive, evaluate, and act in response to the symptoms of disease. While one person will dismiss a particular symptom as not being important, another will seek prompt medical attention. For example, patients who are highly neurotic have a greater tendency to emotional instability and an increased liability to develop abnormal reactions to stressful events; patients who are extroverted are more likely to freely communicate and exaggerate their symptoms. A wide range of sensations: normal physiological functions, benign trivial symptoms, the somatic concomitants of anxiety, as well as the symptoms of serious disease may all be amplified. An amplifying perceptual style may lead to heightened attention to bodily sensations so that a normal irregularity in breast tissue is mistaken for a lump, stomach ache attributed to an ulcer. Such concerns lead to increased apprehension, hypervigilance, and heightened somatic symptoms (Barsky and Wyshak 1990). Obsession with health or ill health may lead to multiple dental visits and demands for further investigation. Decisions to investigate such patients may be influenced as much by the nature of the complaint as by the persistence with which the complaint is reported. A study of patients with backache, for instance, shows that the amount of treatment received was influenced more by the patients' distress than by the actual physical disease

(Waddell *et al.* 1984). So personality factors affect not only patients' decisions to seek medical care but also the type and amount of care they receive. Neuroticism influences the perception of health rather than health itself. Excessive concern leads to a career of hospital attendances, admissions, and investigations to exclude diseases that may account for their symptoms. Somatization, or the physical expression of emotional problems, may also serve an adaptive function in that the stigma of mental stress is avoided.

Interest has grown in the biological basis of personality. De Batista and Glick (1995) have conceptualized personality disorders along symptom clusters. Those most frequently cited are anxiety and inhibition, cognition and perception, impulsivity and aggressiveness, and affective instability. Intriguingly, animal studies suggest a genetic influence on serotonin functioning, which is trait-like and correlates with impulsive behaviour. Serotonin functioning is further influenced by early learning experiences, particularly parental deprivation. Maxillofacial surgeons are likely to encounter much impulsive and aggressive behaviour in trauma victims and an understanding of its genetic basis, combined with the interaction of a vulnerable personality and alcohol or drugs, is important when considering treatment of such patients.

Social circumstances

Social factors modify illness. The strength of social and community supports, such as marriage, contacts with close friends and relatives, church membership, and job satisfaction, all influence not only the onset but also the outcome of psychiatric and physical illness (Brown and Harris 1978). Social circumstances have also been shown to affect such diverse problems as the incidence of pregnancy complications (Nuckolls *et al.* 1972), mortality rate (Berkman and Syme 1979), and the outcome of coronary artery surgery (Grundele 1978). The amount of support available to an individual obviously mediates the effects of any unpleasant life events.

The dental practitioner should always consider a patient's social situation and be sensitive to problems that may arise from a lack of support. Socially isolated patients will place much greater demands on their dentist than those with adequate social contacts.

Evaluation of symptoms by patient and clinician

Symptoms may be discounted as a normal physiological process or interpreted as an indicator of serious disease. Family or individual previous experience of symptoms will make the symptom less threatening and has been shown to diminish motivation to seek medical help

(Banks and Keller 1972). An individual's evaluation is influenced by previous experience, cultural orientation, personality, social support, and mood.

A clinician's evaluation will be modified not only by the history obtained but also by the physician's own personal belief system and psychological characteristics, indeed the success or failure of any treatment may be influenced by this attribute. Emotional tension may arise if the patient feels that his problems are not being taken seriously, if the dentist is in doubt about diagnosis or treatment, or if the patient feels, rightly or wrongly, any antagonism from the practitioner. An individual who is ill, with either physical or psychological problems, has been described as adopting the 'sick role', a position which may free the individual from the usual responsibilities of life at home or at work. Occasionally such protection proves rewarding to patients, who prolong the sick role to defend themselves against taking responsibility in life. Should this happen, the doctor or dentist may need to prevent a breakdown in communication. Dental practitioners should remember that oral manifestations of psychological disorders are not figments of the patient's imagination. Assessment of such patients should include systematic enquiry into what may have happened before the symptoms developed, including life stresses, personality and social factors, and an assessment of why the patient has sought treatment.

COMMUNICATING WITH PATIENTS

Interview techniques

If a patient's symptoms do not respond to a straightforward treatment, a dentist may suspect that a patient's problems may be related to emotional problems, and it is useful to adopt a semi-standardized style of interview. The natural progression of questions from one part of a patient's complaint to another will protect both patient and dentist from unnecessary embarrassment and will also ensure that important areas of a patient's life are discussed. The American Dental Association (1987) encourages dentists to improve communication by listening, making eye contact, having a relaxed body posture, overlooking distractions such as papers or radiographs, sitting with the patient, and answering questions without being defensive. Dentists must not assume that pathology is the exclusive object of therapeutic intervention. It may be important to focus on the dentist–patient interaction, and change professional behaviour to a more relaxed, tolerant, and supportive style. The most common complaint that patients have is that doctors and dentists do not listen to them. Meryn (1998) has suggested better quality of communication in relation to better outcomes for patients. An important part of dentist communication therefore is taking a history.

The American Dental Association (ADA) report stresses that focusing on human relationships rather than technical skills improves patient satisfaction. The dentist is encouraged to listen, even to change the office so that time can be made. Specific recommendations are made in Table 1.1. The ADA also recommended that the more patients know about proposed treatment the better. It is best to sit side by side with a patient to discuss the plan (Table 1.2), without interruptions. The patient must agree to the plan and understand that he takes responsibility for treatment. It is suggested that the following approach is adopted.

History taking

Presenting complaints   Try to define what the patient feels the real problem is. It is useful to ask open-ended questions and to allow the patient time to develop problems. It is important to ensure that the patient believes his problems are being taken seriously and that he is believed. The patient may have more than one presenting complaint, or none at all if under regular dental review, life events may also occur during the course of life-long dental surveillance and treatment. Dentists must remember to attempt to identify medical and social problems in patients they have been seeing for many years.

Table 1.1   Body language for good listening

Skill	
Good eye contact	Represents honesty and self-confidence
Body posture	Open and relaxed to show interest; allow patients to sit upright
Avoid distractions	Do not shuffle papers or read radiographs; give patients your undivided attention
Sit with the patient	Sit down in the patient's presence, shows you are listening
Encourage questions and good communication	Encourage patients to air their concerns; follow-up letters are important
Language and terminology	Speaking skills; ensure that patients understand plans
Staff communication and time	Encourage all staff to be considerate of the patient; do not make patients wait
Office design	Keep the office clean and patient-focused
Personal hygiene	Be aware of your own hygiene
Touch	A light touch on the shoulder will reassure anxious patients

Table 1.2   The treatment plan

Proposed treatment and options

Risks and consequences

Fees

Payment schedule

History of present complaint   It is important to find out how the patient's life, work, appetite, sleep pattern, and concentration have been affected. Often it will be possible for a dentist to make a tentative diagnosis at this point and begin to follow up leads about areas of difficulty in a patient's life.

Past medical history   It is important for a patient with psychiatric problems to be reassured that his problem is being taken seriously— thus a detailed medical and surgical history should be recorded. For instance, the patient with psychogenic pain will be reassured when questioned about other types of psychogenic pain, such as headaches, back, and gut problems, as he will realize that the dentist has some insight into his disorder.

Past psychiatric history   This should be approached cautiously. It is best to ask if the patient has received any treatment for 'nerves' and if any reluctance is shown, the practitioner should withdraw, particularly at the first interview.

Family history   It is important to discover not only if any family members suffered similar problems, which is common in the case of anxiety or pain stress, but also to date the deaths of any close family members, as life events such as bereavement are often associated with the development of neurotic problems and with pain.

Personal history   The dentist should not attempt to detail the whole of a patient's life but an awareness of whether a childhood was happy, schooling completed, work or marriage satisfactory, can give valuable insight into the possible cause of a patient's problem. If emotional topics are discussed, it is sensible for the dentist not to record them until after the interview is finished, as the feeling that 'all this will be on my files' often inhibits patients from revealing their problems freely.

Personal habits   It is important to record any drugs taken, as they can exert effects upon a patient's mental state, for instance β-blockers may cause depression, and also to record alcohol and tobacco intake.

Why seek help now   Ask: 'What worries you most about this? What do you think we should do about this?'

Ending the interview   The dentist should always ask 'Is there anything I have forgotten?' or give the patient room to talk; for instance, 'I have asked an awful lot of questions, is there anything you would like to ask me?' An attempt to explain to the patient what is wrong should be made as simply as possible.

Reassurance

The interview will take time. It is therefore sensible to give an appointment when a practitioner has adequate time available or, if this is impossible to arrange, for the patient to be referred elsewhere. Many dental practitioners may feel reluctant to discuss personal problems because they do not have the appropriate training to deal with them. However, the dentist may well be the person a patient is prepared to place his confidence in and it is important to have some knowledge of how to cope with problems the patients may reveal. For instance, it is important not to leave a patient 'up in the air'—if a problem is disclosed, it should not be ignored but attempts should be made to comment, reassure, and advise the patient as to the most appropriate course of action to deal with the difficulties. It may be helpful to use standardized questionnaires to alert dentists to psychiatric and other problems (Porter and Garman 1989; Feinmann and Zakrewska 1990). General medical practice has benefited enormously from the attachment of counsellors, in the future this may be possible for dentists.

A dentist may feel at this point that referral to a specialist is necessary, and it is important that this decision is made with the patient's understanding and consent. It is vital that the patient is not made to feel that his suffering is imaginary or illness not taken seriously. It is crucial not to say there is nothing wrong to a patient who is obviously in pain. It is important that the dentist understands that his reaction to the patient at these times will shape the patient's capacity to cope with symptoms (see Chapter 6).

Information

Patients want more and better information about their problems and outcome, more openness about the side-effects of treatment, relief of pain, and emotional distress, and advice on what they can do for themselves. Good communication offers tangible benefits in terms of patients' satisfaction and health outcome (Meryn 1998). Maybery and Maybery (1996) have described the importance of ensuring that information fits with the patient's level of literacy, cultural and ethnic background. Consideration should be given to use of audio- and videotapes as well as the written word. Examples of handouts for patients and doctors are given in Appendices 2 and 3.

Consent for treatment

Consent to procedures must be informed and risks acknowledged. Patients must be told if there is more than a 1 per cent chance that they will experience side-effects from a drug. Historically, it was not considered to be in the patients' best interest to tell them the truth about their illness; however, it is now believed that patients have a right to know all aspects of their illness.

Communicating in a research context

As not all patients will wish to take part in research studies, it is crucial to explain that routine treatment will not be affected by taking part in research. Approximately 50 per cent of patients will respond to telephone or postal questionnaires and it may be that patients prefer follow-up by telephone—a recent study indicated that if an enquiry was only about a change of symptoms, 80 per cent of patients would be happy with telephone follow-up (Pal 1998).

MAIN PSYCHIATRIC PROBLEMS

Two approaches to psychiatric diagnosis have been the World Health Organization's (1988) *International classification of disease* (now in its tenth revision, ICD-10) and the *Diagnostic and statistical manual of mental disorders* (now in its fourth revision, DSM-IV) of the American Psychiatric Association (1994). The diagnostic systems are complex; ICD-10, for example, allows 26 varieties of depressive episode, although the American system is more austere, with more rigid criteria. Goldberg and Huxley (1992) have argued persuasively that the taxonomies could be simplified with advantage to health workers and patients.

Goldberg and Huxley (1992) stated that most patients who experience symptoms do so for understandable reasons influenced by the vulnerability of the individual and the magnitude of the impinging stress, 'most people will experience symptoms given sufficient stress—but the degree of stress necessary to release symptoms varies enormously'. They speculate that there are specific links between types of social circumstances and the development of specific disorders.

It is worth considering briefly at this point the ways in which psychiatric disorders present to general dental practitioners. It is important, however, to realize that most psychiatric symptoms occurring in this setting will be mild and often of short duration. It may be better for them to be thought of as distress syndromes that accompany either pain or adverse life events rather than psychiatric illnesses. Emotional disturbance, when present, is often mild and of brief duration, so our present psychiatric classification provides an inadequate measure (Feinmann 1988). Categorical diagnoses are useful in severe mental illness, but are not particularly relevant in less severe illness, where a dimensional model relates social variables to clinical variables (Goldberg 1996).

Psychiatric disorders frequently encountered in the dental practice: definitions and symptoms

These are essentially disorders of adaptation, where the degree of emotion expressed signals a breakdown in normal functioning.

Concept of psychiatric disorder

At the first level, upset and worry may be regarded as the normal and understandable emotional reactions to pain, disability, life-threatening illness, or side-effects of treatment. At the second level, the emotional reaction may be more severe, but has not yet reached the level where it is clearly one of psychiatric disorder, and does not require specific treatment other than a sympathetic ear. At the third level, the disturbance is clearly abnormal, constituting one of the disorders defined below. There are no hard and fast boundaries between these levels, i.e. between what is normal distress, borderline symptom, and pathological disorder. Of the disorders described below, adjustment disorder is the mildest and depressive disorder the most severe.

Adjustment disorder

An adjustment disorder is a marked reaction to an identifiable stress that leads to a change in mood or behaviour that, in turn, leads to impairment of social or occupational functioning. The manifestations include:

- depressed mood, anxiety, worry;
- a feeling of inability to cope, plan ahead, continue in the same situation;
- liability to dramatic behaviour or outbursts of emotion or violence;
- development of bodily symptoms.

None of these symptoms is marked enough to merit a diagnosis of depressive disorder (see below).

The difference between adjustment disorder and depression, is that adjustment disorder does not reach the severity and pervasiveness which would enable it to meet the full specified criteria for depression. An example in dentistry may be the overreaction to a dental procedure or operation. Certain personalities and those who lack social support are especially prone to develop adjustment disorder while in hospital. Those with particularly severe physical illness are also likely to do so. Adjustment disorder may therefore be anticipated in patients in the coronary care unit, or in chronic, disabling disorders, such as diabetes, multiple sclerosis, or cancer, both at the time of initial diagnosis and when coping with relapses.

Anxiety states

These may be acute or chronic and may range from fear to phobic avoidance of routine dental treatment. Anxiety may also either amplify the symptoms of a modest lesion or cause a patient to avoid treatment because of fear of malignancy (see Chapter 2). Excessive anxiety may also occur in patients recovering from operations, but can be prevented by preoperative explanation and reassurance.

Anxiety disorder

For a diagnosis of anxiety disorder to be made, the patient must have experienced the following symptoms over several days:

- apprehension: worries about future misfortunes, feeling 'on edge', difficulty in concentrating;
- motor tension: restless fidgeting, tension headaches, trembling, inability to relax;
- autonomic overactivity: light-headedness, sweating, fast pulse or rapid breathing, abdominal discomfort, dizziness, dry mouth; and/or
- several panic attacks.

A panic attack is a discrete period of apprehension or fear accompanied by at least four of the following symptoms:

- breathlessness;
- palpitations;
- chest pain;
- choking or smothering sensation;
- dizziness or unsteady feelings;
- feelings of unreality;
- tingling of hands or feet;
- hot and cold flushes;
- sweating;
- faintness;
- trembling or shaking.

If the patient experiences these physical symptoms of anxiety during well-defined attacks (usually precipitated by a particular situation, for example leaving the house) the condition is known as 'panic disorder'.

Body dysmorphic disorder

Body dysmorphic disorder (BDD) is defined as a preoccupation with an imagined or minor defect in appearance. In dental patients this may cause patients to be preoccupied with a tooth's appearance or colour or with a smile or a profile. The term 'dysmorphophobia' has also been used in Europe since it was introduced by an Italian Psychiatrist, Morselli, in 1886. In ICD-10, this is diagnosed as hypochondriasis if the belief about a perceived defect is regarded as an overvalued idea. In

DSM-IV, if the belief is a delusion, a patient would receive a diagnosis of 'delusional disorder somatic type' in addition to that of BDD. The diagnosis must have the following symptoms:

- preoccupation or excessive concern with imagined defect;
- clinically significant distress or impairment in function;
- no other accountable mental illness.

Depressive disorder

Diagnosis The diagnosis of depressive disorder requires: consistently depressed mood or loss of interest and pleasure for a minimum of 2 weeks, accompanied by four or more of the following symptoms:

- feelings of worthlessness or guilt;
- loss of energy and fatigue;
- altered appetite and weight;
- retardation or agitation;
- impaired concentration;
- thoughts of suicide;
- changed sleeping pattern.

Depression may be graded as mild, moderate, or severe according to the number of symptoms and the degree of disability they cause (World Health Organization 1992).

Occurrence Depressive illnesses are often preceded by an adverse life event such as bereavement. A typical depressive illness is characterized by biological features such as loss of appetite, disturbance of sleep, lack of libido, and general slowing down of bodily functions, as well as by cognitive abnormalities such as loss of concentration or memory. Fifty per cent of patients who are depressed have pain as their presenting complaint. Furthermore depressed patients may complain they have a foul smell or have a vile taste. However, most depressive illnesses presenting to dentists will not be severe and may show atypical features such as increased appetite and sleep. It is also important to recall that many patients may be unhappy or distressed and that such feelings are not equivalent to severe depression. The dentist may confront such problems in about a third of patients with psychogenic pain and also in situations where the results of treatment are claimed, by the patient, to be unsatisfactory. Patients with malignant disease may also go through a depressive phase as they come to terms with their diagnosis. It is probably sensible for the dentist to refer such patients for specialist help.

Obsessional compulsive disorder

This describes the occurrence of ruminations, rituals of thoughts, which the patient knows to be irrational but which he is unable to resist. This may be reflected in a preoccupation with some normal feature of the oral mucosae, such as the tongue, or by the appearance or contour of restorations or dentures. There may also be an obsessional concern about oral hygiene. These states should be differentiated from body dysmorphic disorder (described in Chapters 4 and 7) in which the patient may have an obsessional concern about his appearance. Patients with obsessional neurosis may respond to reassurance whereas the latter group is more recalcitrant.

Unexplained physical symptoms in the dental clinic: their cause and diagnosis

Patients with bodily symptoms may attend the dentist for several reasons. The symptoms may be explained by recent social stress—people who have recently been bereaved, for example, are known to consult the doctor with a variety of bodily symptoms, including symptoms that cause dental pain. Symptoms may be taken to the dentist because the patient is very worried about having serious organic disease. This also often occurs in the context of recent bereavement (where the fear may be of the same disease that led to the death) or other stress, including marked family or marital conflicts.

Patients who present with somatic symptoms may have no signs of overt distress or psychological symptoms, and do not consider themselves psychiatrically unwell, making a diagnosis of the underlying psychiatric disorder difficult. Such patients do not recognize the connection between the bodily symptoms and the concurrent psychosocial problems, the dentist may need to help the patient make this link.

A number of reasons have been suggested to explain why some patients 'somatize' their depression. For example, the patient may pay selective attention to the bodily symptoms to the exclusion of the psychological symptoms. Alternatively, patients may not wish to disclose their psychological problems, preferring to mention only the bodily symptoms for the dentists to evaluate: dentists can unwittingly reinforce this view if they respond with greater interest to physical symptoms than to psychological symptoms. Such 'differential reinforcement' by the dentist may be echoed by the family, where relatives pay more attention to physical symptoms than to psychological problems. Whereas seeking help from the dentist for physical pain is free of negative connotations, the social stigma attached to psychiatric disorders remains, and underlies the reluctance of some patients to accept, or even discuss, possible psychological reasons for their symptoms.

Some groups are especially likely to present psychological problems in the form of bodily symptoms. Special care is required in the assessment of symptoms in elderly people and people with learning difficulties.

Chronic multiple unexplained symptoms: chronic somatization, somatoform, and conversion disorders

Up to one-fifth of patients who do not have an organic diagnosis are diagnosed as having somatization disorder/hypochondriasis. These are patients who have chronic symptoms in numerous bodily systems that are distressing and disabling but which cannot be explained on the basis of organic disease. Such patients have been referred to as 'thick-file patients', 'heart sink' patients, the 'chronic complainer', and the 'albatross syndrome'.

Although they form a relatively small group, they use a disproportionate amount of health service resources. The main features of somatization disorder are multiple, recurrent, and frequently changing physical symptoms, which have usually been present for several years and are reflected in a long and complicated history of contact with both primary and specialist medical services, during which many negative investigations, or even fruitless operations, may have been carried out. Symptoms may be referred to any part or system of the body, but gastrointestinal conditions (pain, belching, regurgitation, vomiting, nausea, etc.) and abnormal skin conditions (itching, burning, tingling, numbness, soreness, and blotchiness) are among the most common. Sexual and menstrual complaints are also common. The disorder is often associated with long-standing disruption of social, interpersonal, and family behaviour. The disorder is far more common in women than in men and usually starts in early life.

A characteristic feature of this group of disorders is repeated and persistent requests for dental treatment and investigations, in spite of previous negative findings and reassurance by dentists that the symptoms have no physical basis. If any physical disorders are present, they do not explain the nature and extent of the symptoms causing distress and preoccupation of the patient. Even when the onset and continuation of the symptoms bear a close relationship to unpleasant life events or to difficulties or conflicts, the patient usually resists attempts to discuss the possibility of psychological causation; this may even be the case in the presence of obvious depressive and anxiety symptoms. The degree of understanding, either physical or psychological, that can be achieved about the cause of the symptoms is often disappointing and frustrating for both patient and dentist.

Factitious disorder

A few patients present to the dentist with various physical symptoms and signs that are eventually found to be self-induced mucosal lesions, such as ulcers. Patients with factitious disorders who may have been neglected or unwanted as children appear to gain reward by entering and maintaining the sick role.

Patients with factitious disorder are usually aware of the deception involved in their claimed illness, even though the disorder appears to confer no obvious advantage to them. They appear to be driven by underlying psychopathology that drives them to sustain their contrivance, often at considerable risk to their health.

It often transpires that patients have previous experience of organic disease (either in themselves or through working in the medical/nursing sphere) and a personality disorder with pronounced dependent, masochistic, and hostile traits.

Psychoses

A dental practitioner will very rarely be faced by a frankly psychotic patient. The diagnosis is made when the patient loses contact with reality, and is often characterized by delusions (i.e. morbid beliefs out of keeping with the patient's cultural background from which the patient cannot be dissuaded). Briefly, psychoses are divided into:

- the affective psychoses, where depression is characterized by retardation which can be so severe as to cause stupor or profound over-excitement such as mania;
- schizophrenia and paranoid illnesses, which are often characterized by disorders of thinking and delusional ideas which have severe effects on the patient's life.

Personality

Personality traits have been viewed as constitutional and life-long. Eysenck's (1975) original idea of dimensions of stability/neuroticism (N) and intraversion/extroversion (E) has been extended, and a high level of neuroticism is now understood, in terms of complaint behaviour, to be closely related to the number of medical symptoms reported (Katon 1982). In DSM-IV, cluster A personality consists of schizetypal, paranoid, and schizoid personality disorders. Cognitive and perceptual difficulties, problems with interpersonal relationships, or both characterize this group. Group B includes the dramatic and emotional type, which tends to have some difficulties with affective instability and impulsive and aggressive disorders. These include borderline, narcissistic, antisocial, and histrionic personality disorders. Group C includes dependent, avoidant, passive–aggressive, and obsessive personalities. A major feature of these disorders is anxiety and inhibition difficulties.

SUMMARY

It is clear that patients do not develop psychiatric problems in isolation. From the preceding brief review of the effects of stress and social support, it becomes readily apparent that the processes of disease and illness are intimately connected with the life situation and life events in any individual. Both the patient's illness and the medical care received will be determined by the individual personality characteristics, past experiences, current life events, and the presence or absence of social support. It is only by careful enquiry into the antecedents of illness that the different aspects of a patient's illness will be established. The following chapters will be concerned with the details of, and treatment for, such problems.

QUESTIONNAIRES

There are numerous questionnaires to assess psychiatric morbidity. These are summarized and reviewed in Anne Bowling's excellent book, *Measuring disease*.

Psychometric questionnaires

The following questionnaires are most relevant to dentistry. These should not be used in isolation, only after discussion with academic colleagues.

1. Patients' endorsement of pain-coping strategies and pain control can be measured using the 44-item Coping Strategies Questionnaire (CSQ, Rosenstiel and Keefe 1983) which has been used in a multitude of investigations. Reliability and validity have been thoroughly examined.

The authors described a seven-factor solution comprising: reinterpreting pain sensations, increased behavioural activities, diverting attention, coping self-statements, ignoring pain sensations, catastrophizing, and praying and hoping. A two-factor solution of 'active' and 'passive' dimensions has also been described; active coping being related to activity level and passive coping with psychological distress.

2.   Current pain effect and intensity can be recorded by means of the short-form McGill Pain Questionnaire (SF-MPQ, Melzack 1987). This is a valid and reliable instrument for out-patient groups. Both a visual analogue scale (VAS) and a verbal rating scale (VRS) assess present pain intensity. The scale can be used to differentiate different pain groups and to measure change.

3.   The 14-item Hospital Anxiety and Depression scale (HAD, Zigmond and Snaith 1983) assesses mood. A valid and reliable measure of both 'anxious' and 'depressive' symptoms in out-patient populations, the HAD is considered to be free of potentially confounding somatic items. Using psychiatric diagnoses as a gold standard, patients recording anxiety or depression scores of 7 or less are considered to be non-cases, scores of 8–10 are doubtful cases, and scores of 11 or more definite cases. Although such scales do not equate to a psychiatric diagnosis, so-called 'false positives' (i.e. cases according to self-report scales but not to psychiatric interview) have been shown to display greater psychopathology than true negatives, while not differing from true positives on measures of psychosocial dysfunction. However, the HAD may not separate anxiety from depression, and readers who are keen to rate depression and anxiety separately may consider the Beck Depression Inventory Scale (Beck *et al.* 1961) and the Spielberger State/Trait Anxiety Inventory (Spielberger *et al.* 1977).

4.   The 46-item Oral Health Impact Profile (OHIP, Slade and Spencer 1994), which has been developed to assess the social impact of oral disorders. Subscales include physical, psychological, and social disabilities. Its measurement properties have been established in older age groups and modification is needed for younger dentate subjects, by omission of denture-related items.

5.   Beck Depression Inventory (BDI, Beck *et al.* 1961). This 21-item scale was designed to measure severity of depression. It contains affective, cognitive, somatic, and behavioural items.

6.   Spielberger State/Trait Anxiety Inventory (Spielberger *et al.* 1977). This 40-item self-report inventory assesses current subjective feelings of anxiety (state) and more stable, general feelings of anxiety (trait).

7.   Dental fear: the Dental Anxiety Survey (DAS) is established as valid and reliable (Corah 1988).

REFERENCES

Ader, R. (ed.) (1987). *Psychoneuroimmunology*. Academic Press, New York.

American Dental Association (1987). *Risk management manual*. ADA, New York.

American Psychiatric Association (1994). *Diagnostic and statistical manual of mental disorders IV*. American Psychiatric Association, New York.

Banks, F. R. and Keller, M. D. (1972). Symptom experience and health action. *Medical Care*, **9**, 498–502.

Barsky, A. J. and Wyshak, G. (1990). Hypochondriasis and somatosensory amplification. *British Journal of Psychiatry*, **157**, 404–9.

Beck, A., Ward, C., Mendelson, M., and Mack, J. (1961). An inventory for measuring depression. *Archives General Psychiatry*, **4**, 561–71.

Berkman, L. F. and Syme, S. L. (1979). Social networks, host resistance and mortality. *American Journal of Epidemiology*, **109**, 186–204.

Blinkhorn, A. S., Craft, M., Shaw, O., Smith, J., and Speirs, R. L. (1979). Behavioural sciences in the dental curriculum. *British Dental Journal*, **147**, 117–20.

Bowling, A. (1995). *Measuring disease*. Open University Press, Buckingham.

Brown, G. and Harris, T. (1978). *Social origins of depression. A study of psychiatric disorders in women*. Tavistock Publications, London.

Cooper, C. L., Watts, J., and Kelly, M. (1987). Job satisfaction, mental health and job stresses and UK general dental practitioners. *British Dental Journal*, **158**, 77–81.

Corah, N. L. (1988). The dentist–patient relationship—perceived dentist behaviours that reduce patient anxiety and increase satisfaction. *Journal of the American Dental Association*, **116**, 73–6.

De Batista, C. and Glick, I. (1995). Pharmacotherapy of personality disorders. *Current Science*, **8**, 102–5.

Eysenck, H. (1975). *The Eysenck personality questionnaire*. Hodder and Stoughton, London.

Feinmann, C. (1988). The contribution of psychiatry to the understanding of facial pain and headache: problems in diagnosis and management. In: *Headache* (ed. A. Hopkins). Saunders, UK.

Feinmann, C. and Zakrewska, J. (1990). A standard way to measure pain and psychological morbidity in dental practice. *British Dental Journal*, **169**, 337–9.

Ford, C. V. (1983). *The somatising disorders: Illness as a way of life*. Elsevier Biomedical Press, New York.

Goldberg, D. P. (1996). A dimensional model for common mental disorders. *British Journal of Psychiatry*, **168**, (Suppl. 30), 44–9.

Goldberg, D. P. and Blackwell, B. (1970). Psychiatric illness in general practice: a detailed study using new methods of case identification. *British Medical Journal*, **ii**, 439–43.

Goldberg, D. and Huxley, P. (1992). *Common mental disorders*. Tavistock and Routledge Press, London and New York.

Grundele, P. (1978). Recovery from coronary artery surgery. *Heart*, **1**, 1–6.

Holmes, T. H. and Wolff, H. G. (1952). Life situations, emotions and backache. *Psychosomatic Medicine*, **14**, 18–33.

Katon, W. (1982). Depression: somatic symptoms and medical disorders in primary care. *Comprehensive Psychiatry*, **23**, 274–87.

Katon, W. and Gonzales, J. (1994). A review of randomised trials of psychiatric consultation—liaison studies in primary care. *Psychosomatics*, **35**, 268–78.

Katon, W., Von Knorff, M., and Li, E. (1990). Distressed high utilisers of medical care. *General Psychiatry*, **12**, 355–62.

Kent, G. G. (1984). *The psychology of dental care.* John Wright and Sons, Bristol.

Kiecolt-Glaser, J. K. and Glaser, R. (1992). Psychoneuroimmunology. Can psychological interventions modulate immunity? *Journal of Consulting and Clinical Psychology*, **60**, 569–79.

Kroneke, K. and Mangelsdorff, A. D. (1989). Common symptoms in ambulatory care. Evaluation therapy and outcome. *American Journal of Medicine*, **86**, 262–8.

Maybery, J. C. and Maybery, M. (1996). Effective instruction for patients. *Journal of the Royal College of Physicians of London*, **30**, 206–8.

Mechanic, D. (1972). The concept of illness behaviour. *Journal of Chronic Diseases*, **15**, 189–94.

Melzack, R. (1987). The short form MCGMI pain questionnaire. *Pain*, **30**, 191–7.

Meryn, S. (1998). Improving doctor–patient communication. *British Medical Journal*, **316**, 1922–30.

Meyer, R. J. and Haggerty, R. J. (1962). Streptococcal infection in families. *Paediatrics*, **29**, 539–49.

Nuckolls, K. B., Cassel, J., and Kaplan, B. H. (1972). Psychosocial stress, life crisis and the prognosis of pregnancy. *American Journal of Epidemiology*, **95**, 431–41.

Pal, B. (1998). Following up outpatients by telephone: a pilot study. *British Medical Journal*, **316**, 1647–50.

Pilowsky, I. (1969). Abnormal illness behaviour. *British Journal of Medical Psychology*, **42**, 347–51.

Porter, M. and Garman, D. (1989). Approaches to somatisation. *British Medical Journal*, **298**, 1332–3.

Rosenstiel, A. and Keefe, F. (1983). The use of coping strategies in chronic low back pain patients: relationship to patients' characteristics and current adjustment. *Pain*, **17**, 33–44.

Shepherd, J. (1995). Should doctors be more proactive as advocates for victims of violence? *British Medical Journal*, **311**, 1617–21.

Shepherd, M., Cooper, B., Brown, A. C., and Katton, G. (1966). *Psychiatric illness in general practice.* Oxford University Press, London.

Slade, G. D. and Spencer, G. (1994). Development and evaluation of the oral health impact profile. *Community Dental Health*, **11**, 3–11.

Soroway, S. M., Pollack, S., Steinberg, M. D., Weinschel, B., and Malvert, M. (1995). Four year follow up of the influence of psychological comorbidity on medical re-hospitalisation. *American Journal of Psychiatry*, **153**, (3), 397–403.

Spielberger, C. P., Gorsuch, R. L., Luchere, N. (1977). *Manual of the State–Trait Anxiety Inventory.* Consulting Psychological Press, Palo Alto, California.

Tessler, R., Mechanic, D., and Dimond, M. (1976). The effect of psychological distress on physician utilization. *Journal of Health and Social Behaviour*, **17**, 353–64.

Waddell, G., Bircher, M., Finlayson, D., and Main, C. R. (1984). Symptoms and signs: physical disease or illness behaviour. *British Medical Journal*, **289**, 739–41.

World Health Organization (1992). *The ICD 10 classification of mental and behavioural disorders*. WHO, Geneva.

Zigmond, A. and Snaith, P. (1983). The Hospital Anxiety and Depression Scale. *Acta Psychiatrica Scandinavica*, **67**, 361–7.

FURTHER READING

Bowling, A. (1995). *Measuring disease*. Open University Press, Buckingham.

Goldberg, D. and Huxley, P. (1992). Common to mental disorders. Routledge Press.

2

Special problems in dentistry

Charlotte Feinmann and Geir Madland

ANXIETY

Anxiety differs from other emotions in that it is also a drive, a basic motivating force. Anxiety caused by an imminent examination may, for instance, encourage a student to revise or, if the emotion becomes pathological, avoid the feared situation and do no work at all. However, there is a distinction between:

(1) anxiety as a symptom which may be part of everyday experience;
(2) anxiety as a symptom which is a sign of some other illness, such as the anxiety associated with physical illness; and
(3) anxiety which is so severe or of such long duration that it becomes an illness in itself.

Anxiety provoked by dental treatment is a problem for both patients and dental practitioners. It appears to be a normal reaction for individuals to feel some anxiety about dental treatment. Modern dentistry is painless yet fear of pain remains a cause of anxiety. Todd and Walker (1980) interviewed 6000 British residents and found that 43 per cent of the population avoided going to the dentist unless they were in trouble; an attitude which creates conflicts for the dental surgeon who is trained to help the patients and relieve suffering but is regarded by patients as someone who inflicts distress. Kent (1984), in a survey of stresses encountered by dentists in practice found that the most important and common problem was coping with difficult, anxious patients. The situation is complicated, anxious patients expect treatment to be painful, and their anxiety is not modified by a painless experience. Thus coping with anxiety means that patients' preconceptions about treatment must be modified (Bochner 1988).

Presentation of anxiety problems to the dentist

These may vary from a simple overreaction to a dental procedure, to more aggressive responses. Anxious, obsessional, or depressed patients may amplify pain or become agitated after what appears to the dentist to be a normal consultation. Similarly an acute hypochondriacal reaction may be precipitated by an innocent remark or trivial investigation.

The first part of this chapter will deal with how anxiety develops before discussion of the treatment of anxiety.

The development of anxiety

It seems obvious that most people are anxious about dental treatment, because they are anticipating pain. Gale (1972) demonstrated that the amount of fear could not be specified from knowledge of the situation alone and he concluded that a fair amount of dental anxiety was generated about uncertainty about particular treatments. Wardle (1982) asked patients awaiting dental treatment how anxious they felt and how much pain they expected from several dental procedures. She found, not unexpectedly, that highly anxious patients were more fearful of pain. Undoubtedly, previous experience shapes a patient's response to treatment.

Lautch (1971) compared 34 dentally phobic with 34 non-phobic patients and discovered that all of the phobic patients, compared to only 10 of the controls, had had a previous traumatic experience during dental treatment.

The experience of others, particularly close family members, may shape the patient's expectation of dental treatment. Johnson and Baldwin (1968) showed that there was a strong relationship between maternal anxiety and the disruptive behaviour of young children undergoing treatment. However, Koenigsberg and Johnson (1972), in a follow-up study, showed that this relationship did not persist after the patient's first visit, implying that children can learn from reassuring experiences and lose their fear of dental treatment. Such findings are in agreement with the fact that anxiety can result from an abnormal personality trait such as neuroticism. Lautch (1971) found that his dentally phobic patients had higher neuroticism scores on the Eysenck Personality Questionnaire (Eysenck 1975) than the matched samples of non-phobics. Moreover, the dentist can exert a powerful influence on patients' experience. Bernstein et al. (1979) have shown that patients complain of much more anxiety and pain when the dentist is perceived as impersonal, disinterested, uncaring, or cold.

Hallstrom and Halling (1984) examined 784 women, a representative population sample in Gothenburg, and found a prevalence of severe dental anxiety (dental phobia) in 13.4 per cent of the population. Previous studies had found a prevalence rate of between 8 and 15 per cent. The prevalence was much increased in women with low levels of education and in lower social classes. In 88 per cent, the phobia onset occurred before age 20, but only 11 per cent were aware of having been exposed to anxiety-provoking dental treatment prior to the development of phobias. The age of onset is similar to other studies but the lack of a provoking factor is contrary to other work. All studies agree, however, that the disorder runs a chronic course.

Dispositional and coping strategies

It seems that a number of factors contribute to dental anxiety; Fig. 2.1 shows how such anxiety may develop. Uncertainty and fear result from previous learning, which includes the dentist's behaviour, and a biological propensity to develop anxiety and leads to the avoidance of dental treatment. Once this becomes too great, a phobia of dental treatment will develop and the patient will avoid all contact with the dentist. Locus of control, monitoring–blunting, repressing–sensitizing, and high desire to control–low perceived control are dispositional characteristics. Coping skills employed by patients in acute stress situations such as dentistry include distraction, sensory or emotional focus, information seeking, reattribution, and relaxation (Turk and Fior 1987). Maladaptive coping mechanisms include catastrophization, a belief that they will never be able to cope with dentistry.

An individual's dispositional and coping style, combined with mood abnormalities, determine what particular skill will be employed. People benefit from employing coping skills that are consistent with their individual coping style (Litt 1996). Patients with an internal locus of control fared better on self-report measures of pain and distress, following viewing a specific rather than a general information videotape before dental treatment, whereas patients with an external locus fared worse. Litt (1996) in his seminal article suggests there are links between specific strategies and coping styles.

Patient beliefs in relation to seeking dental treatment

It is not only anxiety and fear of pain that prevent patient's attendance. Studies of pain and dental treatment consistently find pain experience is

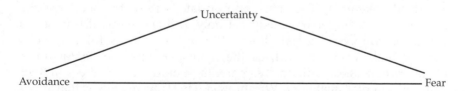

Fig. 2.1 Development of dental anxiety. Fear of dental treatment occurs as a result of uncertainty about the details of treatment and leads to avoidance of such treatment.

less than expected. A large number of individuals do not value their health and attend doctors and dentists only in crisis. Patient beliefs in dentist's abilities and possible benefits from treatment will also determine attendance.

The treatment of dental anxiety

The treatment of the dentally anxious patient is determined not only by the severity of the patient's problem but also the time and training available to the dental practitioner. Behavioural research has developed many techniques designed to desensitize patients with anxiety problems but these may be excessively time-consuming for the average dental surgeon. Ayer (1982) suggested that only 10 per cent of behavioural therapies could be put to practical use in the surgery and stressed the importance of a good dentist/patient relationship in controlling anxiety. Coombs (1980), in a thorough review of the application of such research to the dental setting, suggested that the most important role for the dentist was to be aware of how anxiety problems develop and suggested that prevention of anxiety was possibly a more realistic role for the dentist than cure.

Good prevention

Early fluoridation and improved dental health combined with education about oral hygiene should decrease the possibility of early traumatic experiences and consequent fear of dentistry. There is also increasing evidence that taking children to the dentist at an early age increases their confidence and that the participation of an elder sibling can model good behaviour for them. Ghose *et al.* (1969) showed that four-year-olds were much less disruptive in treatment if they previously viewed elder siblings sitting in a dental chair. Giving adequate explanation of treatment and allowing children to see treatment being carried out also seems to be helpful. Melamed *et al.* (1978) found that showing children films of non-traumatic dental treatment made them less disruptive in later appointments. However, Auerbach and Kilmann (1977) warned that too much information could be aversive to the patient, who would then avoid all treatment. The most appropriate setting for such reassurance and modelling is obviously not only in practice but also in school clinics or children's dental clinics. It may also be useful to involve other dental personnel, such as the hygienists and the dental nurse, at an early stage; additionally, parents should be involved in their children's dental treatment. Wright *et al.* (1973) have shown that modifying maternal anxiety not only improves children's co-operation with dental treatment but improves appointment keeping as well. They stress that a pre-appointment letter explaining what treatment will take place is an important means of gaining a patient's co-operation. Coombs (1980) also suggests that short pre-surgical waiting periods are of value. She found that not only did they prevent anxiety and pain but also reduced recovery periods.

Hallstrom and Halling (1984) suggested, as a result of their findings, that dental phobia develops early in life and runs a chronic course, preventive measures must be directed primarily towards children and adolescents.

The prevention of anxiety in the young is therefore dependent upon the following:

(1) improved dental health;
(2) improved dental education;
(3) the reduction of anticipatory anxiety by modelling and early contact with dentists;
(4) the reduction of maternal anxiety by providing information and accurate times for treatment;
(5) obviously the personality of the dentist is of paramount importance in the success of any of these treatments.

All the evidence suggests that dentists should adopt more explicitly the role of dental health educator. Furthermore, if the dentist becomes responsible for the long-term dental health of the patient he will inspire greater confidence. In so doing, the dentist should also give responsibility to the patient for aspects of maintaining their own dental health. This requires development of patients' understanding as to the causes of dental disease together with strong support, monitoring, and feedback in the area of oral hygiene procedures. A major obstacle to the enlargement of the dentist role identified by Bochner (1988) is the relative infrequency of visits. Bochner suggests that this might be overcome by interspersing conventional dental consultations with sessions devoted purely to educational aims, perhaps conducted in small groups.

The management of moderate anxiety

Once a patient becomes conditioned to fear dentistry, the dentist obviously has to attempt to allay a patient's fears. Mild anxiety may be treated by reassurance, but if this fails, fear of pain can be treated appropriately by adequate pretreatment sedation and analgesia. Pre-medication with a mild tranquillizer such as diazepam has been in use for many years. However, the dental practitioner is increasingly aware of the possibility of addiction with repeated use of such drugs. Pretreatment analgesia has been found to be an effective means of controlling pain. It has the advantage that not only is pain reduced but the experience also becomes a reassuring one for the patient.

Various means of distraction, such as listening to taped music or relaxation tapes (instructions to patients to contract and relax various muscle groups), have been found to be a useful way of alleviating anxiety and pain (Corah *et al.* 1979). Additionally, giving the patient some control over their treatment, such as raising an arm to stop drilling has been shown to be an effective way of reducing anxiety and pain (Wardle 1982). Rankin and Harris (1984) examined a large sample (258) of patients who were not receiving dental care and found that although vicarious and personal experience had made them fear dentistry, it was the fact that they felt unable to cope with the situation that prevented their actually attending appointments. So helping patients to gain control of the situation is obviously an important part of treatment.

The patient's perception of control is often improved by an increased understanding of the treatment. Much of dentistry is amenable to explanation in some detail and a significant proportion of anxious patients are enhanced in their control over treatment by such a process.

The treatment by the individual dentist will obviously depend on his own inclinations as well as the time he has available. Moderate anxiety can then be controlled effectively by the following methods:

(1) reassurance and explanation;
(2) adequate sedation and analgesia;
(3) relaxation;
(4) distraction;
(5) it may be most important to give the patients some control over their treatment.

The management of severe anxiety

The patient who actually manages to attend a dental surgery despite overwhelming anxiety may hopefully be managed by the dentist. This can be done either by treatment with general anaesthetic or, if the dentist is unable or reluctant to provide this, by treatment with intravenous benzodiazepines. General anaesthesia does not increase the perceived control the patient needs to acquire. The use of general anaesthesia limits the time available for the dental procedures to be carried out. It is therefore most suited to disease control and essential dentistry. It should be the aim to move from this to the use of agents such as midazolam. Hall and Edmunson (1983) demonstrated the efficacy of intravenous diazepam in the treatment of 70 phobic patients. Sixty-five were able to complete treatment, two dropped out of treatment, and three patients were rendered edentulous. At a 5-year follow-up of 49 patients, three had had no further treatment, 30 had managed to have treatment under local anaesthetic, and 16 continued treatment with intravenous diazepam.

Hypnosis is also gaining increasing respectability in the management of dental anxiety and pain. Barber (1977) claimed that previous use of hypnosis has been unsuccessful because of the authoritarian attitude of most hypnotists, and he claimed almost 100 per cent success in the control of anxiety and pain with rapid induction analgesia in 100 patients, although Houle *et al.* (1988) found that hypnosis was no better than simple relaxation.

In order to cope with the extremely anxious patient, the general dental practitioner has therefore to use either general anaesthetics, intravenous diazepam, or hypnosis. At present there do not seem to be any other time- and cost-efficient methods available to him in the surgery. Although Lindsay (1996) suggests that dentists should contract with psychologists to provide care, in the present financial situation it is difficult to see how this can be achieved. Berggren and Meynert (1984) studied a large number of phobic patients and found that although patients with isolated dental phobias really benefited from treatment, those with generalized phobias did not.

So it would seem that if the patient is unable to come to the surgery, or if the dental practitioner is unable to cope with him at the surgery, then it is probably necessary to refer the patient either to a hospital where specialized treatment for dental phobias can be given or to a clinical psychologist. The clinical psychologist has a range of skills at his disposal, such as desensitizing the patient to his phobias, providing biofeedback to try and relax the patient, and other methods of relaxation, which, in conjunction with an appropriately motivated dentist, may well be able to provide greater help.

The management of severe anxiety requires:

(1) general anaesthetics;

(2) intravenous sedation;

(3) hypnosis; or

(4) referral to a clinical psychologist.

Summary

In order to manage dental anxiety, it is necessary to understand why that anxiety developed. Most patients are not only frightened of dentists but are also fearful and uncertain about what their dental treatment will be. Prevention of anxiety is important, and to that end improved dental health and improved patient co-operation with treatment are vital. Once anxiety has developed, it is then necessary to attempt to reassure, distract, or sedate the patient, and if all this fails, then either general anaesthetics, intravenous diazepam, or hypnosis should be tried by the general practitioner. Complicated and difficult patients can probably only be treated by referral to a local special needs clinic or to the clinical psychologist.

Several years ago it was recommended in the UK that communication skills be taught in the undergraduate dental curriculum. This has occurred, with great success, in a number of schools but the teaching must continue at a postgraduate level. Communication is an interactive process. Patients will also need skills and support to take part in decision making and to be able to raise questions about care issues (Meryn 1998).

PSYCHOPHYSIOLOGICAL PROBLEMS

Oral ulceration

Aphthous ulcers

Recurrent aphthous ulcers (RAU) occur in 20–50 per cent of the population. This troublesome condition of shallow, painful oral ulcers varies in incidence from sporadic single lesions to recurrent crops. The exact aetiology is unknown, although the condition often has the features of an autoimmune disturbance. Despite this, many patients are aware that emotional problems may precipitate their lesion. For this reason it is useful when patients complain of recurrent crops of painful ulcers to take a full and careful history, including social and emotional factors.

This should be followed up by an ulcer diary, where the patient notes on a day-to-day basis the number of ulcers present in the mouth and any associated factors. Reassurance will often produce a marked reduction in the number, frequency, and duration of the ulcers, making them more amenable to topical steroid therapy.

Factitious ulceration (stomatitis artefacta)

This is the intraoral counterpart of the well-recognized dermatitis artefacta (Sneddon 1977). The lesions will vary in their appearance according to the manner in which they are created. The most common and least troublesome lesion is due to cheek chewing. Here, usually a young, anxious individual continually chews the buccal mucosa, producing wide areas of peeling, macerated, hyperkeratinized epidermis. It is usually bilateral and painless and may be associated with facial arthromyalgia (see Chapter 4). Similarly, lip biting may produce fissures, white areas of hyperkeratosis, or a mucus extravasation cyst. In the older anxious or agitated patient, lip chewing produces varicosities so that the vermilion border becomes curiously cyanotic in appearance.

Greater difficulty may be experienced in recognizing the discrete lesion that local abrasion with a fingernail or sharp instrument may produce. Occasionally, caustic agents such as tablets or undiluted antiseptics may be used. Because of the hysterical element in this condition, the condition may mimic a natural lesion, particularly if the patient is associated with dentistry or medicine. Unfortunately, there appears to be no age, intellectual, or professional barrier to this problem, although women seem to be more prone than men. The history is characteristically vague and the lesion either persists longer or recurs more frequently than one would expect. It is often associated with one of the pain syndromes, and the patient appears to produce the lesion to validate an organic diagnosis for their pain. Sneddon (1977) describes three groups:

(1) true malingerers, where an injury is consciously aggravated for monetary gain or the avoidance of some responsibility;
(2) Münchhausen's syndrome, which is a persistent, incurable psycho-pathic way of life, without any obvious advantage other than obtaining medical and nursing care;
(3) part of an emotional instability, such as a personality disorder, where the underlying problem is a disturbance in personal relationships.

It is rare to obtain an acknowledgement or explanation as to how the lesions are produced, and it is frequently difficult to get the patient or his family to agree to psychiatric help. Nevertheless, this is important in order to protect the patient from inappropriate investigations and treatment.

Anorexia nervosa and bulimia

Anorexia nervosa is pathological avoidance of food where the subject has a delusional body image. Despite emaciation, they see themselves as being fat and, apart from limiting their food intake, there is often a covert practice of vomiting. The bulimic, by self-induced vomiting, maintains a normal weight despite indulging in eating binges. Both groups eventually suffer erosion of their teeth due to the regurgitated acid. The erosion is often severe, affecting predominantly the palatal surfaces of the maxillary teeth, including the palatal cusps of the maxillary posterior teeth. This may produce marked sensitivity to thermal and osmotic stimuli. There is also deterioration in the appearance of the maxillary anterior teeth: there will frequently be chipping of the incisal edges as these are left unsupported by loss of palatal tooth tissue. The incisal edges appear bluer or darker as the teeth become so thin that the darkness of the oral cavity becomes apparent through them. The pattern of wear is highly specific to regurgitated acid. If found on routine examination, the causes of acid regurgitation should be considered in some detail; these will include, in addition to anorexia and bulimia, acid regurgitation due to hiatus hernia or due to chronic alcohol intake. If the acid attack continues for a number of years, sufficient tooth structure may be lost for pulpal vitality to become compromised.

Patients suffering from anorexia and bulimia also tend to have high levels of caries activity. The diet tends to be rich in fermentable carbohydrate and, coupled with low self-esteem which can be reflected in poor oral hygiene procedures, leads to the high incidence of dental caries.

These patients can be very difficult to treat. Their low self-esteem often precludes their entering into treatment. This is unfortunate as the teeth require some form of protection from the gastric acid. This can be in the form of a mouthguard which is coated internally with a small amount of magnesium hydroxide and placed in the mouth prior to vomiting. Patients should also be counselled to refrain from brushing their teeth for three-quarters of an hour after regurgitation, to allow the acid in the mouth to have been dispersed and neutralized. If they can be persuaded to use an aqueous fluoride solution as a mouthrinse, this will be helpful in maintaining the hardness of the teeth. However, the problems of low self-esteem make the motivation difficult.

The damaged teeth generally require restoration if they are to be preserved. Adhesive restorative dentistry has made a significant impact with this type of damage and makes treatment more conservative and less difficult for the patient to receive.

This is a condition where if the opportunity arises to carry out some conservative restoration that will also protect what is left of the teeth, it should be taken, even if the condition is not well controlled.

Treatment requires the close co-operation of the patient, a dietician, a restorative dentist, and a psychiatrist.

Periodontal disease

Chronic inflammatory periodontal disease is caused by bacterial plaque being held in apposition to the gingival tissues. Several investigations suggest a relationship between periodontal disease and emotional conditions. Studies have shown increased anxiety and personality problems in affected patients. Also, individuals exposed to naturally occurring stressful life events have been shown to develop periodontal problems. Various investigations have shown that reduced salivary flow under autonomic nervous system control affects plaque and so causes periodontal problems. Stress may also alter the response of oral tissues to bacterial toxins. Da Silva *et al.* (1997) have conducted studies exploring the mechanism mediating between emotional factors and soft-tissue lesions. Da Silva *et al.* (1995) reviewed the literature and suggested that chronic periodontal disease is affected by psychosocial factors and that the practitioner should take them into consideration and, if necessary, refer the patient for psychological support. In a study of three groups of patients, 50 with rapidly progressive periodontitis (RPP), 50 patients with routine adult periodontitis, and 50 controls with significant periodontal destruction, the RPP patients showed significantly more depression and loneliness than the controls, suggesting the need for an evaluation of psychosocial intervention in this group.

REFERENCES

Auerbach, S. M. and Kilmann, P. R. (1977). Crises intervention: a review of outcome research. *Psychological Bulletin*, **84**, 189–217.

Ayer, W. A. (1982). Dental problems and oral health behaviour. *Journal of Behavioural Medicine*, **4**, 273–95.

Barber, J. (1977). Rapid induction analgesia: a clinical report. *American Journal of Clinical Hypnosis*, **19**, 138–47.

Berggren, U. and Meynert, G. (1984). Dental fear and avoidance: causes, symptoms and consequences. *Journal of the American Dental Association*, **109**, 247–52.

Bernstein, D. A., Kleinkrecht, R. A., and Alexander, L. D. (1979). Antecedents of dental fear. *Journal Public Health and Dentistry*, **139**, 113–24.

Bochner, S. (1988). *The psychology of the dentist–patient relationship*. Springer-Verlag, New York.

Coombs, J. A. (1980). Application of behavioural science research to the dental office setting. *International Dental Journal*, **30**(3), 240–8.

Corah, N. L., Gale, E. N., and Illing, S. J. (1979). The use of relaxation and distraction to reduce psychological stress during dental procedures. *Journal of the American Dental Association*, **98**, 390–4.

Da Silva, M., Newman, H., and Oakley, K. (1995). Psychosocial factors in inflamatory periodontal disease. *Journal of Clinical Periodontology*, **22**, 516–26.

Da Silva, M., Newman, H., and Oakley, K. (1997). Psychosocial factors and tooth wear. *European Journal Prosthodontic and Restorative Dentistry*, **2**, 51–5.

Eysenck, H. J. and Eysenck, S. (1975). *Manual of the Eysenck personality questionnaire*. Hodder and Stoughton, London.

Gale, E. N. (1972). Fears of the dental situation. *Journal of Dental Research*, **51**, 964–6.

Ghose, L., Goddon, D., Shiere, F. *et al.* (1969). Evaluation of sibling support. *Journal of Dentistry in Childhood*, **36**, 35–49.

Hall, N. and Edmunson, H. D. (1983). The aetiology and psychology of dental fear. *British Dental Journal*, **154**, 247–52.

Hallstrom, T. and Halling, A. (1984). Prevalence of dentistry phobia and its relationship to missing teeth, alveolar bone loss and dental care habits in an urban community sample. *Acta Psychiatrica Scandinavica*, **70**, 438–46.

Houle, M. *et al.* (1988). The efficacy of hypnosis and relaxation induced analgesia. *Pain*, **33**, 241–51.

Johnson, R. and Baldwin, D. (1968). Relationship of maternal anxiety to the behaviour of young children undergoing dental extraction. *Journal of Dental Research*, **47**, 801–5.

Kent, G. (1984). *The psychology of dental care*. John Wright & Sons, Bristol.

Koenigsberg, S. R. and Johnson, R. (1972). Child behaviour during sequentional dental visits. *Journal of the American Dental Association*, **85**, 128–32.

Lautch, H. (1971). Dental phobia. *British Journal of Psychiatry*, **119**, 151–8.

Lindsay, S. (1996). Report in *British Medical Journal*, **313**, 189.

Litt, M. P. (1996). A model of pain and anxiety assoicated with acute stresses: stress in dental procedures. *Behavioural Research and Therapy*, **35**, 459–76.

Melamed, B. G., Yurcheson, R., Fleece, E. L. *et al.* (1978). Effects of film modelling on the reduction of anxiety related behaviours. *Journal of Consulting and Clinical Psychology*, **46**, 1357–67.

Meryn, S. (1998). Improving doctor–patient communication. Not an option but a necessity. *British Medical Journal*, **314**, 7149.

Rankin, J. A. and Harris, M. B. (1984). Dental anxiety: the patient's point of view. *Journal of the American Dental Association*, **109**, 43–7.

Sneddon, I. B. (1977). Dermatitis Artefacta. *Proceedings of the Royal Society of Medicine*, **70**, 754–5.

Todd, J. E. and Walker, A. (1980). Adult dental health in England and Wales. HMSO, London.

Turk, D. G. and Fior, H. (1987). Greater than pain behaviours: the utility and limitation of the pain behaviour construct. *Pain*, **313**, 277–95.

Wardle, J. (1982). Fears of dentistry. *British Medical Journal*, **55**, 119–26.

Wright, G. L., Alpern, G. D., and Leake, J. L. (1973). The modifiability of maternal anxiety. *Journal of Dentistry in Childhood*, **40**, 265–71.

FURTHER READING

Cohner, L. K., and Bryant, P. S. (ed.) (1988). *Social sciences and dentistry. A critical bibliography*, Vol. II. Quintessance Publishing, New York.

Kent, G. G. (1984). *The psychology of dental care*. John Wright & Sons, Bristol.

3

Idiopathic orofacial pain: a multidisciplinary problem

Charlotte Feinmann and Richard Ibbetson

DEFINITIONS

Pain is the most common symptom that compels patients to seek medical and dental help, and constitutes a serious health and economic problem. It has been estimated that in the industrialized countries 15–20 per cent of the population have acute pain and between 25 and 30 per cent suffer from chronic pain. This costs American society US$79 billion annually (Bonica 1990).

Dentists and dental specialists are concerned with two of the most common pains. The first being acute orofacial pain arising from the teeth and associated structures and, the second, chronic orofacial pain which is believed to account for 40 per cent of all chronic pain problems. An understanding of the pathophysiology of pain is needed by all those who are involved in pain relief. Table 3.1 gives a summary of the most common pains affecting the mouth and face. The diagnosis of idiopathic orofacial pain is not only one of exclusion, as the diagnosis is made by identifying other problems in the patient's life.

THE PATHOPHYSIOLOGY OF PAIN

Pain is a subjective psychological state rather than an unpleasant sensory activity that is induced solely by noxious stimulation. The definition of pain adopted by the International Association for the Study of Pain (IASP 1986) is 'an unpleasant sensory and emotional experience associated with actual or potential tissue damage or described in terms of such damage'. This definition avoids linking pain to a stimulus and regards pain always as an affective state, that is an emotional experience and not merely the

Table 3.1   Classification of common orofacial pain

Acute	Chronic

Oral
  Dental: pulpits, cracked tooth
 	
  Periodontal: gingivitis, periodontitis,
  pericoronitis
  Mucosal: various cause of ulceration
TMJ: traumatic acute dysfunction
Maxillary sinus: sinusitis and
carcinoma
Salivary glands: acute sialadenitis
Ear: otitis externa
Tonsils: quinsy
Referred: cardiac angina, cervical
spondylosis
	Neurogenic: trigeminal neuralgia
	Nociceptive: cancer, osteoarthritis,
	rheumatoid arthritis
	Chronic and recurrent idiopathic orofacial
	pain:
	  Facial arthromyalgia
	  Atypical facial pain (idiopathic facial pain)
	  Atypical odontalgia
	
	Oral dysaesthesia
	Tension-type headache
	Migraine
	Facial migrainous neuralgia

TMJ, temporomandibular joint.

perception of a pure sensation. However, the affective state of pain differs from other affective states in that it is always referred or projected to some part of the body, with varying degrees of precision (Wyke 1958). Unlike elation or sorrow, pain is always 'felt' in some part of the body, even when that part is no longer present, as in the case when pain is felt in a 'phantom limb' after its amputation.

As pain is a totally subjective experience which can not be simultaneously shared and reported by another individual, it is clinically important to accept the subject's description of the pain experience. Conversely, it is unhelpful to question or reject it.

Acute pain may be a protective mechanism for the body by stimulating the sympathetic nervous system. and anxiety. It is also of considerable diagnostic value to the clinician in determining the nature and site of the disturbance. The control of acute pain in most instances is accomplished by the use of analgesics or surgery. Chronic pain does not serve any apparent biological function and is socially and psychologically destructive. It can be recurrent or continuous. The sympathetic and neuroendocrine responses have usually become less apparent and vegetative (somatic) signs emerge similar to those seen in depressive syndromes (Sternbach 1981). Furthermore, its control is invariably achieved by specific forms of medication, such as anticonvulsants for trigeminal neuralgia, ergotamine for migraine, and tricyclic antidepressants for chronic idiopathic pain as well as for the prophylaxis of migraine.

PAIN MODULATION

The concept of pain modulation is based on the evidence that neural impulses are altered as they travel up to the higher centres.

It has been traditional to divide pain into organic and psychogenic. Organic being pain that has resulted from an identifiable structural lesion, while psychogenic not only labelled those pains without such a lesion but also implied a 'supratentorial' psychiatric disturbance. Emphasis has changed to the main factors that influence the excitation and inhibition of the painful experience. Whether the pain is generated by a noxious stimulation of the tissues or occurs as a result of a central affective disturbance is no longer of great concern. Pain is regarded as a sensory and emotional experience that always involves structural changes somewhere in the body.

Melzack and Wall proposed their 'gate-control' theory to explain the variability of the painful experience. Later, based on new information, they modified this theory (Melzack and Wall 1982). These theories have proved to be among the most important developments in the field of pain research and therapy. In addition to providing a comprehensive formulation of pain mechanisms, they have stimulated much physiological and psychological research and provoked the development of new approaches to pain therapy.

The pain-modulating network

There appears to be a specific central nervous network for pain control. Analgesia may be demonstrated by stimulation of brain sites such as the periaqueductal grey (PAG) and nucleus raphe magnus (NRM) in animals and humans. This has provided powerful evidence for highly selective brainstem control of nociceptive transmission (Fields and Heinricher 1985). This system is also involved in emotional and motivational functions and other complex behaviour.

Although there has been much emphasis on the pain-suppressing effect of the modulation system, the brainstem-modulating neurones have a bidirectional control of transmission in that the network has both excitatory and inhibitory actions on pain conduction. These concepts are incorporated in the new model of the gate-control theory. Therefore pain can result from either the loss of inhibitory control or the activation of excitatory modulating neurones.

Recently, a quantitative study of regional cerebral responses to non-painful and painful thermal stimuli in six atypical facial patients and six matched female controls was performed by monitoring serial measurements of regional blood flow by positron emission tomography (PET)

(Derbyshire *et al.* 1994). Both groups displayed highly significant responses to painful heat in the thalamus, anterior cingulate cortex, caudate nucleus, insula, and prefrontal cortex. These structures are closely related to the medial pain system. The atypical facial pain group shared greater activation of anterior cingulate cortex and lesser activation of prefrontal cortex. These differing activations may be responsible for the maintenance of chronic pain through the failure of inhibition of other cortical and limbic structures.

The anatomical, chemical, and physiological bases of pain modulation are progressively being unravelled. Analgesia produced by the pain-modulating network is believed to be mediated by endogenous opioid substances that are synthesized by nerve cells and have pharmacological properties nearly identical to those of narcotic analgesic drugs. The first-discovered endogenous opioid peptides were leucine enkephalin and methionine enkephalin (Hughes *et al.* 1975). Since their discovery, other opioid peptides have been identified throughout the body. One of the most potent of these is β-endorphin ('endogenous morphine'). Its precursor, pro-opiomelanocortin, which originates in the infundibular nucleus of the basal hypothalamus, also gives rise to adrenocortico-trophic hormone (ACTH). However, it is interesting that ACTH antagonizes the analgesic effects of β-endorphin. This may also be of some relevance to chronic pain conditions, as patients with chronic idiopathic pain syndromes are reported to have higher levels of cortisol in their blood (Blumer *et al.* 1982).

Cytochemical studies of the pain-modulating networks have also revealed that in addition to the endogenous opioid peptides, several other neurotransmitters are involved in the control of pain transmission. The monoamines, serotonin and noradrenaline, are present in the brainstem neurones and both inhibit spinal cord pain transmission cells (Basbaum *et al.* 1983; Yaksh 1983).

The endogenous opioid system and the monoaminergic network interact, and recent studies have shown that morphine may activate the descending serotoninergic pathway and so modulate dental pain transmission (Yonehera *et al.* 1990).

Monoamines have also been implicated in the pathogenesis of chronic pain and are of particular importance as they can be manipulated by a variety of pharmacological agents, thus raising the possibility of new centrally acting analgesic agents. In fact there is evidence that the well-established value of tricyclic antidepressants in chronic pain management (Feinmann and Harris 1984) relates to their potency as blockers of the reuptake of both noradrenaline and serotonin (Taiwo *et al.* 1990; Botney and Fields 1983).

The use of antidepressants as analgesics opens up an entirely new approach to drug treatment for chronic pain. These drugs do not produce tolerance and dependence and their side-effects have been considerably diminished with the development of novel agents.

PHYSIOLOGICAL BASIS OF TREATMENT

A biochemical basis for chronic facial pain was suggested by the association with depression and the response to tricyclic antidepressants. Magni (1987) also found a high percentage of emotional disorders in first-degree relatives of chronic pain patients. However, the relief of pain by tricyclic antidepressants occurs just as effectively in non-depressed, psychiatrically normal patients.

We now have evidence that the 'facial pain patient' is biochemically vulnerable and can be identified by a reduced urinary excretion of conjugated tyramine sulphate, which also happens to be found in patients with endogenous depression (Aghabeigi *et al.* 1993). Furthermore, tricyclic antidepressant medication has been thought to increase midbrain serotonin levels, which are concerned with central analgesia (Von Knorring *et al.* 1978).

CHRONIC IDIOPATHIC FACIAL PAIN

Chronic idiopathic facial pain (CIFP) is a common problem. More than 10 million Americans suffer chronic pain in the face at a cost to society of over US$4 billion a year, and between 25 and 45 per cent of the population are affected at some time in life (Bonica 1990; Lipton *et al.* 1993; Von Knorff 1996). A recent National Institutes of Health Report (NIH 1996) stated that CIFP is a collection of medical and dental conditions affecting the temporomandibular joint (TMJ) and/or muscles of mastication as well as the face, mouth, and teeth. There is an absence of clear guidelines for diagnosis and management, and many practitioners attempt therapy with new and inadequately tested methods.

Box 3.1   Chronic idiopathic facial pain

- Ten million affected in the USA.
- Severity variable.
- Who should be treated?
- What constitutes treatment?

The age range for facial pain extends from childhood to late adult life, with peaks at 30 and 50 years (Feinmann and Harris 1984*a*). It is three times more common in females than males, although some claim that men are equally affected but many more women seek treatment, emphasizing the importance of consulting behaviour.

It is not known how many patients improve without treatment. Nor is it clear, other than from patients' requests, what types of symptoms, signs, and other assessments provide a basis for indicating therapeutic interventions. Numerous assessment methods are available, but lack of evidence of the diagnostic value of these tools means that diagnosis often depends on the practitioners' experience and philosophy rather than scientific advice. The severity may vary from clinically insignificant to seriously debilitating pain.

Furthermore, there is no consensus on the validity or relevance of the various diagnoses (Feinmann and Bass 1989; Marbach 1995), which are based on signs and symptoms rather than aetiology. Dworkin and Leresche's (1992) research diagnostic criteria represent a very reasonable start. The criteria have a biaxial approach, with carefully integrated specified physical factors with comparable specifications of psychological status. They are, however, rather extensive; what is needed is the development of clinical guidelines and some evidence that the diagnostic criteria have clinical utility. Woolf *et al.* (1998) have suggested a mechanism-based classification of pain, with operational criteria, inclusion and exclusion criteria, and validity. Validity is defined with reference to a gold standard, the absence of which is a challenge in headache and pain classification.

The various diagnoses include tension headaches, migraine, neck-aches, facial arthromyalgia, (temporomandibular joint dysfunction), and atypical (idiopathic) facial pain. These pains differ from trigeminal neuralgia in that they appear to arise from blood vessels, muscles, and joint capsules rather than as primary disturbances of sensory nerves.

Unfortunately, these disorders tend to be separated by artificial distinctions in clinical presentation, so that some patients with pain thought to be arising from joints and muscles are treated by dental specialists, and others by neurologists, otorhinologists, and psychiatrists, with little collaboration between the specialities, except for referral to offload the patient to the next speciality. The American Academy of Orofacial Pain (Rosenbaum *et al.* 1997) has recently concluded that CIFP should be diagnosed and treated in a manner consistent with the diagnosis and treatment of any system of joints and muscles in the body—head and neck pain management rather than TMJ management.

There are additional important problems concerning the recognition and definition of underlying psychiatric disturbances. Emotional disturbance, when present, is often mild and of brief duration and so our present psychiatric classification provides an inadequate measure (Williams *et al.* 1980; Feinmann and Bass 1989). Often the undergraduate curriculum does not assist in recognition of the disorders. Medical students receive no training in dentistry nor do dental students receive any significant training in psychiatry. Graduates in either speciality are therefore ill-equipped to recognize many facets of the disorders in which facial pain and headache are prominent symptoms. That chronic somatic symptoms reflect emotional disturbances is often overlooked (Katon *et al.* 1990).

The recognition of latent emotional disturbance can benefit both the individual and the health services. Early recognition and treatment of emotional disturbance may prevent the symptoms from becoming intractable. The recognition of psychological factors may prevent unnecessary investigation and costly intervention, including further consultations with other hospital specialists. (Katon *et al.* 1990).

There is a pressing need to reach a common agreement on a unifying classification of chronic idiopathic orofacial pain associated with emotional disturbance. Currently, different professional specialities concerned with the treatment of these patients still advocate opposing aetiological theories, ranging from pure mechanical malfunction to emotional distress, with consequent confusion to the patient and treatment. This chapter will review the various orofacial symptoms. Chapter 4 will assess the role of the orofacial specialist, the liaison psychiatrist, and the psychologist in managing this difficult patient group.

Clinical features

Four symptom complexes are recognizable: facial arthromyalgia (FAM) (i.e. temporomandibular joint pain dysfunction syndrome; myofascial pain dysfunction syndrome), atypical facial pain, atypical odontalgia, and oral dysaesthesia (Feinmann and Harris 1984). Although perceived to be separate conditions, they often coexist or occur sequentially in the same patient. Given the uncertain aetiology and the considerable overlap in symptoms with the conditions that produce pain in and around the area of the temporomandibular joint, many authors may prefer to adopt the term temporomandibular dysfunction (TMD) (Okeson 1996) which does not ascribe a particular aetiology to the condition. The term does not, however, include other facial pains—so the term chronic idiopathic orofacial pain is used in this text.

Facial arthromyalgia

Symptoms vary from a clicking, uncomfortable jaw joint on chewing, talking, and yawning to a continuous dull ache with severe exacerbations often described as earache. The pain radiates widely to the masseteric, temporal, occipital, and mastoid areas or down into the neck (Fig. 3.1). It rarely seems to prevent or disturb sleep. The patient is often troubled for many weeks or even intermittently for many years. He may also give a history of headaches, disturbed hearing, fullness, popping, or tinnitus in the ear. There appears to be a strong clinical association with other symptoms.

Bruxism (clenching and grinding of the teeth) is one form of parafunction, and other oral habits include nail, pencil, or pipe biting, and cheek or lip chewing. These, or other forms, are commonly found whether or not there is FAM, although the patient may not be aware of such activity when first asked.

Aetiology

Two principal concepts have dominated the clinical scene in various forms: (1) the occlusal (Krogh-Poulsen and Olsson 1966) and (2) the psychophysiological (Laskin 1969).

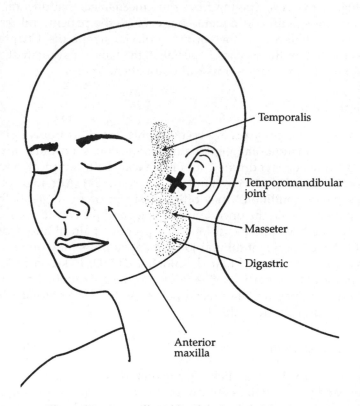

Figure 3.1   Areas affected by chronic orofacial pain

Box 3.2 Facial arthromyalgia

FAM includes:

- pain in the face, jaw joint;
- headaches;
- earaches;
- dizziness;
- masticatory muscle hypertrophy;
- limited opening;
- clicking or popping in the joint.

It should now be accepted, despite strong traditional beliefs, that there is no evidence that malocclusion will give rise to this chronic pain disorder (Carlsson and Droukas 1984). The incidence of malocclusion is no higher in patients with FAM than in the general population (Thomson 1971) and, surprisingly, there is no published study showing that occlusal correction is more effective than placebo adjustment or simple counselling (Kopp 1979). Also, the dominantly female susceptibility calls into question any simplistic theory of occlusal disharmony. On the other hand, there is such evidence that stress, adverse life events, and vulnerable personality types predispose to the condition (Feinmann and Harris 1984; Speculand *et al.* 1984). Yemm (1992) has also elegantly reviewed the research showing that central neuromuscular control gives rise to muscle hyperactivity, bruxism, and joint overloading, rather than local reflex disturbances. Griffiths (1983) stated in an ADA workshop on TMJ disorders that 'it is legally bad practice to link malocclusion with TMD in our own mind or in a patient's'.

Clinical assessment

A conventional medical history and examination reveals that FAM is part of a widespread pain syndrome in many patients. These patients may also suffer locally, atypical facial pain (a chronic non-muscular, non-joint facial pain), atypical odontalgia, and oral dysaesthesia. More remotely, they have tension headaches, neck and back pain, irritable colon, pruritus, and dysmenorrhoea (Feinmann and Harris 1984), all conditions which can have a strong psychological background.

Differential diagnosis

A small but distinct group of patients presents with joint pain and dysfunction following an acute or chronic history of trauma. The many possible causes of this internal derangement include extraction of wisdom teeth or tonsillectomy under general anaesthesia, competitive swimming, singing, whiplash injuries of the neck, or as a late complication of ipsi- or contralateral joint trauma or surgery.

The history is usually free of stress-related features, and where joint noise or pain and limitation of opening persist, there is invariably evidence of intracapsular damage on tomography and arthrography. These patients should be classified as traumatic TMJ derangements or, where appropriate, especially in the elderly, osteoarthrosis.

A full blood count, erythrocyte sedimentation rate (ESR), and serology tests for rheumatoid arthritis may be considered necessary in some cases.

Atypical facial pain (atypical facial neuralgia, idiopathic facial pain)

There is debate concerning the value of atypical facial pain (AFP) as a distinct diagnosis, but it is a common form of pain which is usually described as a continuous dull ache, with intermittent excruciating throbbing episodes that are localized to a non-muscular site such as the alveolar bone or over the maxillary antrum. The pain may be bilateral with a wide extrafacial distribution and is not provoked by jaw movements and rarely relieved by analgesics. Occasionally there is a strong resemblance to facial migrainous neuralgia with a sensation of nasal stuffiness or obstruction; the pain waking the patient in the early hours of the morning. Bouts of pain may last for hours or days and the patient may have a history of intermittent pain over a period of many years.

A common feature is that the pain may be provoked or potentiated by trauma or dental treatment. In the older, edentulous case, the patient cannot wear one or both dentures despite bone smoothing procedures and the provision of innumerable prostheses with and without soft linings. Apart from occasional marked hyperaemia of the oral mucosa or slight oedema of the face, there are no clinical signs.

Ruth Moulton (1966) used the term 'atypical facial pain' to describe what was thought to be an hysterical conversion syndrome; this is undoubtedly rare. Lascelles (1966) felt that these patients were suffering from depression. However, Feinmann and Harris (1984) showed that AFP patients did not differ from the FAM patients in their psychiatric morbidity or socio-demographic characteristics. This is not surprising as the symptom complexes are not mutually exclusive and may occur sequentially or simultaneously in the same patient. However, Harrison *et al.* (1997) found that as a group AFP patients were more disabled and

---

Box 3.3 Atypical facial pain

Symptoms include:

- dull ache;
- intermittent severe pain;
- non-muscular;
- often bilateral.

---

more psychologically distressed than FAM patients. This may have reflected a longer history of pain. The patient often displays certain recognizable characteristics, such as an obsessive but dependent personality, has inadequate support from parents or spouse, or extreme protectiveness or guilt in relation to a child who may have some congenital problem such as epilepsy or cleft palate. The pain is exacerbated at times when these close relationships are disturbed by illness or death. For these reasons the examination and history are as described in the section on FAM.

Pain mechanism

The pain mechanism appears to be vascular and the patient often suffers from other pains with a muscular or migrainous quality, which may include neck, shoulder, and back pain, and may also have a history of peptic ulceration, irritable bowel, dysmenorrhoea, menorrhagia, or pruritis.

It has been argued that AFP may be a form of deafferentation pain or represents a heterogeneous group of idiopathic pains, including the postviral fatigue syndrome. For these reasons, the term 'atypical facial pain' has been declared unfashionable by the International Association for the Study of Pain. (Merskey 1986). However, this doctrinaire approach is clinically unhelpful, particularly without an alternative designation and also because the recommended drug therapy (see below) has proven invaluable in most cases.

In some patients, a paroxysmal trigeminal neuralgia can provoke a more continuous atypical facial neuralgia component, possibly due to a reactionary depression resulting from the primary neuralgia. If this accompanies the tic, the clinician may erroneously assume that the neuralgia has become uncontrollable and requires surgery, whereas the therapy should include an antidepressant drug in addition to carba-mazepine. One also encounters the occasional trigeminal neuralgia which suddenly changes its character from an intermittent paroxysmal pain controlled by carbamazepine to a more continuous pain responding only to antidepressant drugs. Again, these patients have a background of significant emotional disturbance.

Differential diagnosis

Although a primary diagnosis can be made on the recognition of this history and presentation, it is crucial to exclude other causes of facial pain, such as dental caries, sinus disease. and nasopharyngeal and intracranial tumours. This not only necessitates a careful clinical examination including the cranial nerves and appropriate radiographs, but also a computed tomography (CT) scan of the head is essential if there is any suggestion of impaired sensation or motor function. The possibility of a latent neoplasm or intracranial aneurysm, although rare, should also be continually borne in mind on subsequent follow-up, even if the pain remits during drug therapy. A hybrid combination of atypical facial pain and trigeminal neuralgia may also be the first indication of demyelination prior to multiple sclerosis. Chronic, ill-defined facial pain with a muscle and joint component and generalized malaise is sometimes diagnosed as myalgic encephalomyelitis (postviral fatigue syndrome).

Tension-type headache/primary daily headache

Tension-type headache, or perhaps more correctly, primary daily headache, is a steady, non-pulsatile, band-like ache which may be acute or chronic. The pain radiates to the forehead, temples, back of the head and neck. It may be uni- or bilateral and may involve the temporal, occipital, or parietal regions or a combination of all these areas.

The continuous character may be interrupted by pounding exacerbations associated with nausea and vomiting and photophobia. This presentation is often misdiagnosed as migraine. The acute form is very common and affects both sexes equally; however, with the chronic form, four times as many women present for diagnosis and treatment. The condition is associated with stress, anxiety, and depression. The exclusion of hypertension and intracranial lesions is, of course, essential in making such a diagnosis.

It had been assumed that the pain occurred as a result of muscular contraction. However, Phillips (1978) questioned the traditional assumption that these headaches are caused by sustained contraction of the skeletal muscles of the shoulders, neck, and head. She found considerable overlap between EMG records during headache and non-headache periods and suggested that other changes besides muscular spasm affected the presence or absence of head pain (Phillips and Hunter 1981). These could be vascular or central nervous system disturbances. Simple analgesics are used for acute cases, but recurrent chronic cases can be controlled with tricyclic antidepressants. In some patients, supportive psychotherapy and cognitive therapy can be effective.

The commonly observed relationship of FAM and AFP with head pains has led to the belief that malocclusion is not only responsible for FAM but also migraine. However, there is no good evidence for this hypothesis. Furthermore, although 38 per cent of FAM patients have tension headaches, there is no significant association of FAM with migraine (Watts 1986).

Atypical odontalgia (idiopathic periodontalgia, phantom tooth pain)

Odontalgia is usually due to infective or traumatic inflammation of the pulp or periodontal membrane, but patients may present with identical symptoms without any discernible cause (Harris 1974). The pain is severe and throbbing in character and the teeth are hypersensitive to any stimulus. It is often widespread and bilateral but occasionally may be precisely localized.

Box 3.4   Atypical odontalgia

Symptoms:

- severe throbbing pain;
- hypersensitive to all stimuli.

Some cases have been precipitated by a dental procedure such as the fitting of a bridge or the extraction of a tooth. They are not resolved by further dental treatment and in many instances are made worse. One is confronted by a patient with a history of pain accelerated by unnecessary pulp extirpations and extractions and whose remaining teeth, even when sound and vital, are tender to percussion.

The problem appears to be an idiopathic state of hyperalgesia of the pulp and/or periodontal pain receptors. A carefully taken history will reveal significant emotional problems in many patients, and the condition may arise after a period of depression, especially where drug therapy has ceased or as part of the so-called 'postviral fatigue syndrome'. Others may not manifest the features of a primary psychiatric disorder and, as in some cases of atypical facial neuralgia, attempts to force such a diagnosis on them do not produce any therapeutic advantage. Occasionally, hypotensive drug therapy may precipitate the condition, suggesting that a disturbance in catecholamine metabolism may be an important aetiological factor. These patients are best considered to have a variant of atypical facial pain and should be treated in the same manner. The temptation to devitalize or extract teeth must be strenuously resisted.

The condition has been considered to be a deafferentation neuralgia (causalgia) arising when a dental extraction or pulp extirpation produces either an amputation neuroma or a central degenerative change in the trigeminal nucleus. This is an attractive explanation, except that many cases arise without a history of extraction or pulp extirpation, and with pain that may migrate across the midline. Atypical odontalgias are not consistently abolished with a dental local analgesic block. Attempts to curette or excise microscopic neuromas invariably have little effect beyond 1–2 weeks.

However, repeated root canal therapy and local surgery could well produce a causalgia which complicates both the aetiology and clinical features.

Intractable pain

Although this is an apparently arbitrary classification, there is a residue of patients in the previously mentioned groups whose symptoms either persist indefinitely or recur sufficiently often for them to be considered separately.

The study of what Pilowsky and Spence (1976) have called an abnormal illness behaviour sheds some light on why patients suffer from long-standing and intractable symptoms. They suggest that with many conditions 'patients' form a very small group compared to the individuals in the general population who may be shown to suffer similar symptoms. This need to attend a doctor or dental surgeon has been described as the taking up of the 'sick role', and the process leading up to it has been called by Mechanic (1972) 'illness behaviour'. Physical symptoms may be the end result of many kinds of distress due to social and cultural pressures, life events involving real or symbolic losses, marital discord, etc. The illness is presented by the patient for the doctor's diagnosis, which endorses the sick role for the individual, his family, and for society. The usual pattern once such an illness has been diagnosed is for the symptoms to respond to explanation, reassurance, and other appropriate treatment. When the patient does not respond then this may be described as 'abnormal illness behaviour'.

One advantage of Pilowsky's approach is that it seeks to avoid pejorative labelling, such as calling the patient a malingerer, hypochondriacal, or hysterical. It also involves the recognition of the full range of complex factors that lead to the patient presenting with facial pain, emphasizing the importance of taking a comprehensive history which goes into the patient's background and seeks to understand this lack of normal response (Marbach *et al.* 1988). Such an understanding may lead to appropriate conservative (i.e. non-surgical) management of the intractable patient, with attention being paid to previously untreated factors.

Curiously enough, patients with refractory pain are often relatively uncomplaining and appear to be satisfied with continued consultations (if sufficiently long and supportive) in which the same unchanging symptoms are discussed and treatment is prescribed. However, Sternbach (1974) describes these refractory cases as playing 'pain games', where the patient derives some form of benefit from the persistent pain, and has suggested that these benefits include financial compensation, narcotic analgesics, or even the satisfaction of baffling the clinician. Some of such patients could be classified as suffering from hysteria, which is best considered to be a state where the illness represents an unconscious means of attracting emotional support or evading responsibility. The pain or dysaesthesia is thus a peripheral symptom of an underlying psychopathological conflict, and for this reason is called a conversion symptom.

The only clues to the diagnosis are the length of suffering, and a previous history of questionable surgical procedures, especially when associated with personal or family crises. Vigorous attempts to deprive some of these patients of their symptoms may even precipitate a crisis such as dramatic syncopal attacks, urinary retention, whole-body analgesia or ataxia, all without detectable neurological cause and which remit as suddenly as they arise. Lefer (1966) has noted the precipitation of frank psychotic states in such patients following vigorous 'anti-pain treatment'.

The concept of untreatable non-malignant pain is difficult to accept, especially by surgeons. Despite this, any temptation to operate should be resisted, especially as most procedures not only result in irreversible damage but also appear to contribute to the intractability (Gershman *et al.* 1977). For pain 'crises' a regimen of simple analgesics supplemented with an antidepressant drug appears to be an effective means of management, if the patient will tolerate continued medication and the clinician continued complaints of pain.

Psychotic pain

Despite the fact that these pains ultimately appear to be either delusions or hallucinations, on first presentation they have no special qualitative characteristics. The distinguishing clinical features are to be detected in the behaviour of the patient, whose story invariably contains unusually vivid or bizarre details and whose visit is often followed later by a long letter. Paranoid elements seem to be an essential feature—dentists, doctors, relations, or religious and racial groups have all contributed to the patient's suffering.

Such patients seek support from their Members of Parliament and Community Health Councils, who unwittingly collude with their complaints. Occasionally the patient manifests the incongruous emotional reactions of schizophrenia, and discrete questioning usually reveals previous psychiatric treatment and a family history of instability. Care must be taken in examining putative lesions, which are usually factitious, that is, self-inflicted with either a fingernail, needles, or a corrosive agent such as aspirin, an undiluted antiseptic, or a household cleansing agent.

Rarely one encounters the more florid Münchhausen's syndrome, where the patient skilfully and repeatedly induces unwary surgeons to carry out operations for delusional symptoms which may include pain (Oldham 1974). Antipsychotic drugs, such as trifluoperazine and haloperidol, and psychiatric supervision are essential.

Myalgic encephalomyelitis (the postviral fatigue syndrome, Royal Free disease, Icelandic disease, epidemic neurasthenia)

Some patients with AFP or FAM have been given a diagnosis of postviral fatigue syndrome. This is a perplexing syndrome of chronic disability presumed to follow a virus infection. In many cases there is little resemblance to the syndrome, whereas other patients have many of its recognizable features, including a history of infectious mononucleosis.

Characteristic features of the illness (RCP 1997) include low-grade fever, headache, blurred vision and/or diplopia, stiff neck, vertigo with a positive Romberg test, nausea, vomiting, lymphadenopathy, emotional lability, insomnia and/or vivid dreams, frequency or retention of urine, and varying degrees of deafness or hyperacusis. Most cases have a history of a respiratory or gastrointestinal infection, but instead of an uneventful recovery there is persistent and profound fatigue. Muscle fatigue is perhaps the characteristic symptom of the disease and the diagnosis should not be entertained without it.

The most common explanation is that the illness represents an abnormal response to various trigger viruses such as the Epstein–Barr virus, coxsackie group B virus, and subacute myelo-optic neuropathy virus (SMON). There is no treatment and the validity of the diagnosis is not yet proven. Unfortunately, the diagnosis may be given to patients with a long-standing history of unrecognized depression with multiple somatic symptoms.

Oral dysaesthesia (disturbance of oral sensation)

There are several common disturbances in oral sensation, which may occur singly or together:

- the burning tongue (glossopyrosis, glossodynia);
- denture intolerance;
- disturbance in taste (dysgeusia) and salivation;
- the phantom bite syndrome.

The burning tongue

The most common presentation of this condition is the burning tongue, which has been called glossopyrosis or glossodynia. Occasionally the gingiva and lips are also involved or the denture-bearing areas of the hard palate and lower alveolus, making the wearing of a denture impossible.

The patient is often middle aged and female but can be any age or either sex. The picture is invariably one of a burning sensation that gradually increases in severity and frequency until the patient suffers it for the greater part of every day. It may present on waking and very quickly builds up to its maximum intensity for that day. It may be unilateral or bilateral. The most striking feature of the condition is that it is usually relieved by eating or drinking and patients may chew gum or other food in order to seek relief. Other pains of the tongue are made worse by eating and drinking and this distinction may be crucial in making the diagnosis.

The patient's greatest concern is the fear of cancer, and occasionally the appearance of the tongue supports this fear. Patients express concern about the normal appearance of the circumvallate papillae at the junction between the anterior two-thirds of the tongue and the posterior third. Others may be worried about a slightly furred tongue with scalloped margins produced by parafunctional activity against the molar teeth. There is very little evidence to relate these symptoms to any abnormality.

Denture intolerance

Denture intolerance due to discomfort or pain in the absence of any mucosal or bony lesion is a comparable problem. The diagnosis can be made from the many sets of dentures carried by the patient.

A common presentation is with posturing of the jaw and bizarre complaints such as an inability to speak clearly. Most studies of this condition appear to reveal a high percentage of patients with psychogenic or idiopathic denture intolerance.

A full history and appropriate investigations should eliminate any deficiencies of serum iron, vitamins B_{12}, B_1, $B_{2>}$, and B_6, and folate. A localized diabetic neuropathy can be excluded by blood and urine glucose estimations. Candidiasis, unless clinically obvious, does not appear to be a causative factor, but it is probably worthwhile carrying out acrylic patch tests where there is mucosal inflammation. This leaves the bulk of these patients to be classified as either psychogenic or idiopathic. Both should be treated with antidepressant drug therapy.

Disturbances in taste and salivation

The persistent 'nasty' taste, usually with an obsessional concern of having halitosis, and the dry mouth sensation may occur separately or together with a burning tongue. This patient may also complain of dysphagia. Examination invariably reveals no gross oral, pharyngeal, or antral sepsis. Where the complaint is principally that of a dry mouth, there may be adequate or overtly reduced salivary flow. However, sialography and salivary gland biopsy and stimulated flow rates to exclude Sjögren's syndrome are normal. Further, concern in patients over halitosis is not uncommon. It is important to establish not only good toothbrushing but also effective cleaning of the aproximal surfaces of the teeth. Patients should also be advised about the avoidance of spicy foods.

Variations include an illusion of sand in the saliva, excess saliva, or excess mucus, which cannot be objectively substantiated.

These complaints are often a manifestation of stress. Recognizable causes are professional worries, bereavement, loneliness and, curiously enough, in women, the premature retirement of a successful husband (perhaps a symbolical bereavement). The patient may also show symptoms of agitation, early waking, loss of appetite and libido. There is occasionally a firmly held delusional explanation such as amalgam fillings, 'hyperacidity', or impaired pancreatic or hepatic function, which makes the problem a monosymptomatic hypochondriacal psychosis. The clinician often has to compete with a homeopathic practitioner in treating the patient, and a natural remission due to the combined reassurance of both medical worlds is invariably attributed to the latter! More bizarre features are seen with psychotic personalities who may blame contaminated or poisoned food or drink.

Patients with insight and a short history often respond dramatically to explanation and reassurance, or a short course of an antidepressant drug. Long-established cases may be experiencing a marked phase of depression which will require intensive psychiatric therapy. If neglected, the combination of depression, oral discomfort, and dysphagia may lead to a fatal anorexia.

The phantom bite syndrome

Although not uncommon, this problem was probably first described by Marbach (1978). These patients complain of continuous discomfort because their teeth do not meet correctly.

They are often intensively involved with, and superficially knowledgeable about, details of dental anatomy, physiology, and restorative dentistry. At consultation they frequently present numerous radiographs of the teeth, casts, splints, old crowns, and pictures of themselves when perfect. A careful history will reveal a long succession of attempted treatment plans by a variety of dentists who have not been successful. The spouse may be involved in the delusion (a *follie à deux*). Dentists must be cautious in trying to provide any treatment for these patients.

The same applies to removable prostheses and one wonders if, in such cases, the presentation may even be an emotional response to the traumatic loss of the patient's natural dentition. This pathological narcissism is comparable to other phantom syndromes where a limb or breast has been removed. Psychogenic orofacial problems even appear to follow mutilating surgery elsewhere in the body. Like some cases of oral dysaesthesia, this condition has the characteristic features of a monosymptomatic hypochondriacal psychosis.

It is possible that the problem is a disturbance in kinesthesia (position sense), particularly as this can be produced experimentally when vibration is applied to muscle tendons (Goodwin *et al.* 1977). Prolonged dental treatment, especially occlusal equilibration and the replacement of natural tooth contour, may have a similar effect, especially in obsessional individuals. Continued attempts to 'equilibrate' the occlusion do not help.

If there is no clinical evidence of an iatrogenic grossly deranged occlusion, the condition should be considered to be an obsessional or psychotic problem. If this is not recognized, the patient will eventually be rendered cuspless, then edentulous, incapable of tolerating false dentures and invariably acquiring other intractable syndromes.

These patients may be reasonably easy to diagnose if the condition has been present for a number of years. The history of unsatisfactory restorative work, if reported by the patient and investigated by the dentist, will be helpful, but the history of dissatisfaction and discomfort is sometimes very plausible. Dentists should remember that it is unusual for people to be particularly concerned about the detail of how their teeth occlude.

There has traditionally been a great emphasis in restorative dentistry on the accuracy of the occlusion: this is no less so today. However, the main reasons for this are to control the loads on restorations and to stabilize the position of the teeth, there is little to connect occlusal discrepancies with temporomandibular dysfunction. Much interest has centred on the discrepancy between the position of the mandible on closure into the intercuspal position as compared with the retruded axis position. For many years, it was considered that this could be a source of discomfort to patients. This emphasis has now lessened and although the retruded axis position makes a convenient mandibulo-maxillary relationship for extensive restorative work, it does not necessarily confer any physiological benefit on the patient. It is therefore prudent to consider what the approach should be for someone who complains that their occlusion is wrong or that the functional shape of a restored tooth is incorrect.

If the diagnosis of phantom bite is in doubt, their response to a full-coverage maxillary, or occasionally mandibular, occlusal splint should be assessed. This provides a reversible way of providing the patient with an ideal occlusion, albeit in plastic. If the problem is one relating to the occlusion, the splint kept in adjustment should be capable of relieving the patient's discomfort. If this cannot be achieved, the problem is extremely unlikely to be occlusally related.

As with BDD (body dysmorphophobic disorder), patients are usually very certain as to the nature of the problem and are not tolerant of a delay in restorative intervention. It is therefore essential that the dentist considers the assessment and diagnosis carefully, rather than allowing the patient to direct the nature and pace of any treatment.

These patients usually refuse to see psychiatrists and are not amenable to psychotherapy. Fluoxetine 20 mg daily is sometimes helpful but it is difficult to persuade the patients to take the tablets. Without medication the disorder is often intractable and the patient litigious. The American Association of Victims of Dentistry, a self-help organization designed to help patients with 'post orthodontic iatrogenic injury' should be a warning to all dentists to be cautious when planning treatment.

Anything but minimal intervention is bound to fail and the patient will reject the dentist and move on to further help. Co-treatment by psychiatrist and dentist can be successful.

Associated symptoms: physical

It is crucial for an understanding of these patients to realize that headache and facial pain are not the patient's exclusive problems. Nor are these symptoms mutually exclusive, as they may occur sequentially or simultaneously in any patient. Eighty per cent of patients will complain, if prompted, of other recurrent symptoms, such as chronic neck and low back pain, migraine, pruritic skin disturbances, irritable bowel, or dysfunctional uterine bleeding. (Feinmann and Harris 1984). The

---

Box 3.5   Quest for the perfect bite

1. Patient seeks help.
2. Patient praises dentist.
3. Dentist offers help.
4. Patient rejects bite.
5. Dentist rejects patient.
6. Patient sues dentist.

---

prevalence of these symptoms is much higher than in the general population, indicating that facial pain and headache are features of a more generalized somatization disorder. The range of symptoms, however, may not be elicited by specialists unfamiliar with variety of the disorders.

There does not seem to be an adequate muscular correlate to account for the pain of tension headache or facial arthromyalgia (Oleson and Jenson 1990), and there is not a satisfactory explanation about the aetiology of atypical facial pain. The combination of a number of disorders may be a manifestation of what has been termed a 'vulnerable neurochemistry' or a pain-prone patient (Engel 1959; Katon *et al.* 1990; Aghabeghi 1996).

REFERENCES

Aghabeigi, B., Feinmann, C., Glover, V. *et al.* (1993). Tyramine conjunctions deficit in patients with chronic idiopathic temporomandibular joint and orofacial pain. *Pain*, **54**, 159–63.

Basbaum, A. I., Moss, M. S., and Glazer, E. J. (1983). Opiate and stimulation produced analgesia: The contribution of the monamines. *Advances in Pain Research Therapy*, **5**, 323–39.

Blumer, D., Zorick, F., Helibronn, M., and Roth, T. (1982). Biological markers for depression in chronic pain. *Journal of Nervous and Mental Disorders*, **170**, 425–8.

Bonica, J. J. (1990). General considerations of chronic pain. In *The management of pain*, (ed. J. J. Bonica), pp. 180–3. Lea and Febiger, International Association for the Study of Pain, Philadelphia.

Botney, M. and Fields, H. L. (1983). Amitriptyline potentiates morphine analgesia by a direct action on the central nervous system. *Annals of Neurology*, **13**, 160–4.

Carlsson, G. E. and Droukas, B. (1984). Dental occlusion and the health of the masticatory system. *Journal of Craniomandibular Practice*, **2**, 141–5.

Clayton, J. A. and Beard, C. R. (1982). Effect of occlusal splint therapy on TMJ dysfunction. *Journal of Prosthetic Dentistry*, **44**, 324–35.

Derbyshire, S. W. E., Jones, A. K. P., Derain, P., and Feinmann, C. (1994). Cerebral responses to pain in patients with atypical facial pain measured by positron emission tomography. *Journal of Neurosurgery and Psychiatry*, **57**, 1166–72.

Dworkin, S. F. and Leresche, L. (1992). Research diagnostic criteria for temporomandibular disorders. *Journal of Craniomandibular and Orofacial Pain*, **6**, 301–50.

Engel, S. L. (1959). Psychogenic pain and the pain prone patient. *American Journal of Medicine*, **26**, 899–918.

Feinmann, C. and Bass, C. (1989). The limitations of psychiatric diagnosis in the management of chronic pain. In Human psychopharmacology, (ed. P. Stonier and I. Hinuarch), Vol. 2, pp. 219–34. Wiley, Chichester.

Feinmann, C. and Harris, M. (1984). Psychogenic facial pain management and prognosis. Part 1 The clinical presentation. *British Dental Journal*, **156**, 205–8.

Fields, H. L. and Heinricher, M. M. (1985). Anatomy and physiology of a nociceptive modulatory system. Philosophical Transcript Royal Society of London. *Biology*, **308**, 361–74.

Gershman, J. A., Burrows, G. D., and Reade, P. C. (1977). Orofacial pain. *Australian Family Physician*, **6**, 1219–25.

Goodwin, F. K., Cowdry, R. J., Immerson, P., *et al.* (1977). Serotonin and noradrenalin subgroups in depression; metabolite findings and clinical pharmacology correlations. APA.

Griffiths, R. H. (1983). Report on the president's conference on the examination, diagnosis and management of TMJ disorders. *Journal of the American Dental Association*, **106**, 75–7.

Harris, M. (1974). Psychogenic aspects of facial pain. *British Dental Journal*, **136**, 199–202.

Harrison, S., Glover, L., Feinman, C., *et al.* (1997). A comparison of antidepressant medication alone and in conjunction with cognitive behaviour therapy for chronic idiopathic facial pain. In *Proceedings of the 8th World Congress on Pain*, (ed. T. Jesson and J. A. Turner), p. 663. ASP Press, Seattle.

Hughes, J. A., Smith, T. W., Kisterlitz, K. H. W., *et al.* (1975). Identification of two related peulapeptides from the brain with potent opiate agonist activity. *Nature*, **258**, 577–9.

IASP (1986). *International Association for the Study of Pain, Subcommittee on Taxonomy: Classification of chronic pain*, Vol. 3, p. 217. IASP Press, Seattle.

Katon, W., Von Korff, M., Lin, E. *et al.* (1990). Distressed high utilizer of medical care. *General Hospital Psychiatry*, **12**, 355–62.

Kopp, S. (1979). Short term evaluation of counselling and occlusal adjustment in patients with mandibular dysfunction involving the TMJ. *Journal of Oral Rehabilitation*, **6**, 1–9.

Krogh-Poulsen, W. G. and Olssen, A. (1966). Occlusal disharmony and dysfunction of the stomabgnathic system. *Dental Clinics of North America*, **10**, 627–35.

Lascelles, R. G. (1966). Atypical facial pain and depression. *British Journal of Psychiatry*, **112**, 651–9.

Laskin, D. M. (1969). Aetiology of the pain dysfunction syndrome. *Journal of the American Dental Association*, **85**, 892–5.

Lefer, L. (1966). A psychoanalytic view of a dental phenomenon. *Contemporary Psychoanalysis*, **2**, 135–6.

Lipton, J. A., Ship, J. A., Larach Robinson, D. (1993). Estimated prevalence of reported orofacial pain and dysfunction in the US. *Journal of the American Dental Association*, **124**, 115–21.

Magni, G. (1987). On the relationship between chronic pain and depression where there is no organic lesion. *Pain*, **31**, 1–21.

Marbach, J. (1978). Phantom bite syndrome. *American Journal of Psychiatry*, **135**, (4), 476–9.

Marbach, J. (1995). Reaction to Chapters 12 and 13. In *Temporomandibular disorders and related pain conditions: Progress in pain research and management*, (ed. B. Sessel, P. S. Bryant, and R. A. Dionne), Vol. 4, 245. IASP Press, Seattle.

Marbach, J., Lennon, M. C., and Dohrenwend, B. (1988). Candidate risk factors for temporomandibular pain and dysfunction syndrome: psychosocial, health behaviour, physical illness and injury. *Pain*, **34**, 189–51.

Mechanic, O. (1972). Social psychological factors affecting the presentation of bodily complaints. *New England Journal of Medicine*, **286**, 1132–9.

Melzack, R. and Wall, P. D. (1982). *The challenge of pain*. Basic Books, New York.

Merskey, H. (ed.) (1986). Classification of chronic pain: description of chronic pain syndromes and definition of pain terms. *Pain*, (Suppl. 3), 1–90.

Moulton, R. (1966). Emotional factors in non-organic temporomandibular joint pain. *Dental Clinics of North America*, **10**, 609–24.

Okeson, J. P. (1996). *Orofacial pain. Guidelines for assessment, diagnosis and management*. The American Academy of Orofacial Pain. Quintessence Books, USA.

Oldham, L. (1974). Facial pain as a presentation in Von Munchausen's syndrome. *British Journal of Oral Surgery*, **12**, 86–90.

Olesen, J. and Jensen, R. (1991). Getting away from simple muscle contraction as a mechanism of tension-type headache. *Pain*, **46**, 123–4.

Phillips, C. (1978). Tension headache: theoretical problems. *Behaviour, Research and Therapy*, **16**, 249–61.

Phillips, C. and Hunter, M. (1981). The treatment of tension headache: E.M.G. normality and relaxation. *Behaviour Research and Therapy*, **19**, 499–507.

Pilowsky, I. and Spence, N. D. (1976). Illness behaviour syndromes associated with intractable pain. *Pain*, **2**, 61–71.

Ramfjord, S. P. and Ash, M. M. Jr (1995). *Occlusion*, (4th edn). W. B. Saunders, Philadelphia.

RCP (1997). *Report on chronic fatigue*. Royal College of Physicians, London.

Rosenbaum, R. S., Gross, S. G., Perteo, R. A., *et al.* (1997). The scope of TMD/orofacial pain (head and neck pain management) in contemporary dental practice. *Journal of Orofacial Pain*, **11**, (1), 78–82.

Speculand, B., Hughes, A. O., and Gross, A. N. (1984). The role of stressful life experience in the onset of temporomandibular joint dysfunction pain. *Community Dentistry and Oral Epidemiology*, **12**, 197–202.

Sternbach, R. A. (1974). *Pain patients' traits and treatments*. Academic Press, New York.

Sternbach, R. A. (1981). Chronic pain as a disease entity. *Triangle Sandoz*, **20**, 27–32.

Taiwo, U., Fabian, A., Pazoles, C., and Fields, H. L. (1990). Further studies on the mechanism of the potentation of morphine antinociception of monoamine uptake inhibitors. *Pain*, **21**, 329–38.

Thomson, H. (1971). Mandibular dysfunction syndrome. *British Dental Journal*, **130**, 187–93.

Von Knorring, L., Almay, B. C. L., Johanon, G. *et al.* (1978). Pain perception and endorphin levels in CSF. *Pain*, **5**, 359–85.

Von Knorff, M. (1996). Health services research and temporomandibular pain. In *Progress in pain research and management*, (ed. B. J. Sessle, P. S. Bryant, and R. A. Dionne), Vol. 4, p. 227. IASP Press, Seattle.

Watts, P. (1986). Migraine and temporomandibular joint pain. The final answer. *British Dental Journal*, **161**, 170–95.

Williams, P., Tarnopolsky, A., and Tiand, D. (1980). Case definition and case identification in psychiatric epidemiology. *Psychological Medicine*, **10**, 101–14.

Woolfe, C., Bennett, G., Doherty, M. *et al.* (1998). Towards a mechanism based classification of pain. *Pain*, **77**, 227–29.

Wyke, B. D. (1958). The surgical physiology of facial pain. *British Dental Journal*, **104**, (5), 153–68.

Yaksh, T. L. (1983). Direct evidence that spinal serotonin and noradrenaline terminals mediate the spinal antinociceptive effects of morphine in periaqueductal gray. *Brain Research*, **60**, 180–5.

Yemm, K. (1992). The structure and function of the temporomandibular joint. *British Dental Journal*, **173**, 127–32.

Yonehara, N., Shibutani, T., Imai, Y., and Inoki, R. (1990). Involvement of descending monaminergic systems in the transmission of dental pain in the trigeminal nucleus caudalis of the rabbit. *Brain Research*, **508**, 234–40.

4

Chronic idiopathic orofacial pain

Charlotte Feinmann, Richard Ibbetson, and Geir Madland

FACTORS INFLUENCING CLINIC PRESENTATION AND MANAGEMENT

Epidemiology

Over the past decade there has been an increasing awareness that there is a much greater incidence of orofacial pain than patient referral might suggest. In addition, when populations are studied in the clinic, women usually outnumber men by three to one, but the ratio is lower in the general population. Headache and orofacial pain are not unique in having a high prevalence and a low incidence (Lipton *et al.* 1993). It appears that there is a large 'symptom iceberg' for many psychological and physical illnesses, suggesting that the decision to consult a doctor or a dentist is not simply a question of the presence of symptoms. The decision to consult may be to do with symptom severity in combination with complex psychological and social influences. Awareness of changed bodily function occurs frequently in the general population but perhaps only one-third of symptoms are differentially liable to lead to consultations. For instance, Banks and Kellner (1971) found that people were more likely to see their doctor with sore throats than headaches. Clearly, there are several factors, such as fear of cancer or exposure to illness in the family, and many intermediate steps which may be involved in the decision to seek help.

Severity of symptoms

One of the most obvious reasons why some sufferers with headache and facial pain might choose to consult while others do not is the severity of their symptoms. However, a basic problem in interpreting the results of many epidemiological studies is that most investigators have monitored only the presence or absence of symptoms; severity is rarely measured. Heloe *et al.* (1980), in a comparison of patients with facial pain and dental controls, found that consulting groups were more likely to consider their symptoms severe and to take steps to relieve them than others. An individual's own perception of the severity and meaning of symptoms initiates a cycle of distress–appraisal–action (Fig. 4.1).

Appraisal involving first self, then family members and other acquaintances precedes medical consultation. Evaluation of a symptom will be modified by each interaction. An individual will therefore either discount a headache or pain in the face as unimportant, or will interpret such symptoms as a sign of more serious illness, dependent upon his own previous experience and the previous experience of his social contact. Furthermore, the clinician's pain beliefs will determine the nature and the extent of investigation and treatment and may therefore directly affect the outcome of treatment (Kellner 1986). Surgeons will cut, dentists drill, and physicians prescribe carbamazepine given the same presentation. Hottof (1998) has shown an increased incidence of abdominal pain in childhood in adults who develop multiple somatic symptoms. The authors suggest that the medical profession must be alert to the dangers of increasing pain behaviours, relating excessive attention in childhood to later pain behaviours.

Unfortunately the chronicity of these patients and their unrecognized psychogenic features may lead to many patients being offloaded or abandoned. This was reflected in a formal audit of 800 new referrals to the Maxillofacial Department at the Eastman Dental Hospital in an

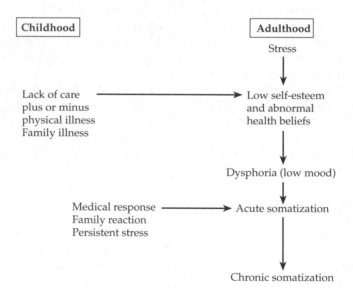

Fig. 4.1   An aetiological model of functional somatic symptoms: the transition from acute to chronic somatization.

18-month period. Their mean pain duration was 4.2 years (median: 1–2 years) despite having been seen by an average of two consultants. At least 25 per cent were tertiary referrals to the department and the cost to the health agencies was immense. Furthermore, many patients had symptoms of such severity that they felt unable to work.

Associated personality and psychiatric problems

There is no consistent evidence that patients with facial pain have a characteristic personality profile, although sufferers may be more compulsive than healthy controls. Furthermore, the concept of a long-standing and relatively immutable personality structure exerting a major influence on disability and outcome treatment is simplistic. Costa and Macrae (1985) have shown that the personality dimension of neuroticism is systematically related to the number of medical symptoms reported. Thus complaints related to neuroticism are a reflection of the amplification of bodily concern. Some people persistently under report medical symptoms, others display more overt somatization.

Somatization is used here to describe the process by which patients communicate emotional distress in concern about physical symptoms and seeking help for them (Katon *et al.* 1990). Somatization may present in the form of anxious 'hypochondriacal concern of developing a disease' or non-anxious 'conviction of having a disease'. These patterns will probably reflect two ends of a continuum of psychiatric disturbance. The psychological state of an individual may induce pain, increase the severity with which it is felt, or even diminish the severity. The patient experiences pain, which may be the only outlet for emotional distress, and the symptoms are often attributed to a physical cause. The disorders are difficult to classify psychiatrically, but the various classification systems attempt to classify somatizers according to symptom, sign, and course with varying degrees of success.

There have been several attempts to examine the psychological status of facial pain patients. These are reviewed in Tables 4.1–4.4. The International Classification of Disease 10th Review (ICD-10) is probably the most simple to apply in practice. However, it is difficult for patients to understand terms such as 'persistent somatoform pain disorder'. It may be more appropriate to describe the physical signs and symptoms of pain.

In comparison with other chronic pain groups, facial pain patients have the lowest rate of psychological illness. A study of 51 patients with a diagnosis of temporomandibular disorder, found that over 50 per cent failed to satisfy the DSM-IV criteria (American Psychiatric Association 1994) for major or minor depression. However, this sample was taken from a specialist facial pain clinic and therefore may not be representative of facial arthromyalgia (FAM) sufferers as a whole.

A community study of 780 individuals found a greater prevalence of clinical symptoms of FAM in depressed women than in non-depressed women, according to a self-rating scale. A further study of acute and chronic FAM, using the structure clinical interview for DSM-III-R

Table 4.1 Comparison of the three main schedules in diagnosing emotional aspects of pain

Characteristic symptoms and signs	ICD-10	DSM-IV	IASP
Preoccupation with chronic pain No organic pathology or gross disparity between examination findings and illness behaviour	Persistent somatoform pain disorder	Pain disorder(associated with psychological factors and/or general medical condition)	Monosymptomatic
Belief of definite disease	Hypochondriacal disorder	Hypochondriasis	Hypochondriacal subtype
Multiple symptoms (<12) from at least two different symptoms of the body	Somatization disorder	Somatization disorder	Multiple complaints
Depressive symptoms Severe depression with delusions of disease, death, or deserved punishment	Depressive episode Severe depressive episode with psychotic symptoms	Dysthymia Major depressive episode Major depressive episode with psychotic features	Pain associated with depression
Delusions of physical defect, disorder, or disease	Delusional disorder	Delusional disorder (somatic type)	Delusional or hallucinatory pain
Pain due to persistent muscle contraction	Psychological factors associated with diseases	Physiological factors affecting physical condition	Muscle tension pain

DSM-IV, *Diagnostic and Statistical Manual*, 4th edn; IASP, International Association for the Study of Pain; ICD, International Classification of Pain.

Table 4.2   Studies that have investigated facial pain patients

Author	Sample	Design	Diagnosis (physical)	Other	Results
Vimpari et al. (1995)	780 community subjects	Correlational	TMJ sounds, limited opening, self reported pain	ZSDS	Subjective and objective symptoms of FAM more common in depressed subjects
Zautra et al. (1995)	110 female myofascial face pain	Longitudinal	Tenderness in muscle(s) of mastication; TMJ sounds or limited opening over 12 months	Two in-person and 10 telephone interviews; over 12 months	Pain and distress stable across months: 'trait' components correlated; Increases in monthly reports of pain preceded by elevated psychological distress in previous month
Korszun et al. (1996)	72 chronic facial pain patients	Correlational	Pain diagnosis from history, clinical, and radiographic examination	DSM-IV, single psychiatrist	53% major/minor depression; 22% depressive symptom
Gatchel et al. (1996)	50 chronic and 51 acute; TMDS's (> or <6 months)	Correlational	RDC/TMD	SCID for DSM-III-R	Both groups showed greater than normal lifetime and current prevalences of psychopathology; acute groups showed higher rates of anxiety disorders and lower rates of affective disorders than chronic group

DSM-III-R, *Diagnostic and Statistical Manual*, 3rd edn, Revised; DSM-IV, *Diagnostic and Statistical Manual*, 4th edn; FAM, facial arthromyalgia; RDC/TMD, Research Diagnostic Criteria for Temporomandibular Dysfunction; SCID, Standardized Clinical Interview for Depression; TMD, temporomandibular dysfunction; TMJ, temporomandibular joint; ZSDS, Zung's Self-rating Depression Scale.

Table 4.3   Studies that have investigated depression in chronic pain patients

Author	Sample	Design	Measures	Other	Results
Brown (1990)	243 RA patients	Longitudinal (seven 6-monthly waves of data collection)	CES-D	AIMS Pain; VAS	Higher levels of depressive symptoms than controls. Pain predicts depression (last 12 months)
Magni *et al.* (1994)	2324 community subjects	Longitudinal (two surveys 7 years apart)	CES-D	Self-reported pain	Odds ratio for pain predicting depression larger than vice versa
Goldberg (1994)	201 chronic pain patients (various)	Correlational	BDI	IASP pain classification; interview re. childhood history	Positive relationship between depression and history of childhood sexual and physical abuse
Turk *et al.* (1995)	100 chronic pain patients (mostly back)	Correlational	CES-D	MPI; ODI	Pain–depression association stronger in older patients (>70 years)

AIMS Pain, Pain scale of Arthritis Impact Measurement Scales; BDI, Beck Depression Inventory; CES-D, Center for Epidemiological Studies, Depression Scale; IASP, International Association for the Study of Pain; MPI, West HavenYale Multidimensional Pain Inventory; ODI, Oswestry Disability Index; RA, rheumatoid arthritis; VAS, visual analogue scale.

(*Diagnostic and Statistical Manual*, 3rd edn, revised), found anxiety disorders in nearly 50 per cent; acute, somatoform disorders in half; and affective disorders in a third of chronic patients.

There is a long-standing association in the literature between atypical facial pain (AFP) and psychological distress, particularly depression. There is plenty of evidence for a high prevalence of anxious and depressive symptoms in oral dysnaethesia patients (44–92 per cent). These studies have not always used standardized measures, but among the methods used are structured interview and self-report scales. However, no longitudinal study has been undertaken to establish the nature of the temporal relationship between psychological factors and oral dysaesthesia patients.

Table 4.4 Studies that have investigated anxiety in chronic pain patients

Author	Sample	Design	Measures of anxiety	Other	Results
Dworkin *et al.* (1992)	19 acute herpes zoster patients	Longitudinal	STAI	MPQ, BDI, LSES, DAS, ASQ, IBQ, SRE	Patients who develop chronic pain had, for example, initially higher trait and state anxiety
McCracken *et al.* (1993)	43 low back pain patients	Longitudinal	PASS	Pain prediction during SLR test, anxiety experienced (0100)	High pain-anxious subjects reported greater pain and experienced anxiety; low-pain anxiety subjects underpredicted pain
Casten *et al.* (1995)	479 geriatric institutionalized subjects	Correlational	DSM-III-R, POMS	Pain intensity and frequency (15)	Anxiety/pain and depression/pain relationships exist even when controlling for strong correlation between anxiety and depression
Morley and Pallin (1995)	100 chronic pain patients (CLBP, RA, headache and controls)	Correlational	HAD	MPQ, CSQ verbal descriptor similarity judgement task	Anxiety differed between groups: CLBP > headache > RA > controls

ASQ, Attributional Style Questionnaire; BDI, Beck Depression Inventory; CLBP, chronic low back pain; CSQ, Coping Strategies Questionnaire; DAS, Dysfunctional Attitude Scale; DSM-III-R, *Diagnostic and Statistical Manual*, 3rd edn, Revised; HAD, Hospital Anxiety and Depression Scale; IBQ, Illness Beliefs Questionnaire; LSES, Life Satisfaction in the Elderly Scale; MPQ, McGill Pain Questionnaire; PASS, Pain Anxiety Symptoms Scale; POMS, Profile of Mood States; RA, rheumatoid arthritis; SLR, straight leg raising test; SRE, Schedule of Recent Experiences; STAI, StateTrait Anxiety Index (Spielberger).

Depression in chronic pain

The prevalence of depression in chronic pain populations is 10–100 per cent. The size of this range is due to several methodological problems inherent in assessment studies, including disparate diagnostic methods, sample selections, overlap of symptoms of pain and depression (sleep disturbance, change of appetite, fatigability, loss of libido) on measurement scales, and lack of prospective studies. The prevalence of depressive symptoms in chronic pain groups is, however, consistently higher than in the general population and many other medical populations (Ramano and Turner 1985).

The psychiatric classification criteria for depression are syndromal (for example, DSM-IV 1994). Diagnoses are defined as syndromes, comprising combinations of affective, cognitive, and somatic–vegetative signs, and symptoms of depression. In addition, a certain duration and other inclusion and exclusion criteria are specified.

There is little evidence for a greater prevalence of syndromal depression in chronic facial pain patients relative to the general population; depressive symptoms being much more common than the major syndrome of depression. A new diathesis–stress framework (Banks and Kerns 1996) encourages identification of vulnerability factors in the individual as well as investigation into the nature of stress. Other research that has concentrated on coping has demonstrated that adaptive coping strategies yield better adjustment and maladaptive strategies worse adjustment (Feinmann and Madland 1998). This concept is developed in Chapter 6.

Box 4.1 An understanding of psychological distress in orofacial pain patients suggests three groups of patients (Feinmann and Bass 1989)

- The emotionally fit individual under stress.
- Those with transient emotional illness such as anxiety or depression.
- Those with a personality trait towards hypochondriasis which persists throughout life.

It is important to emphasize that the majority of patients do not merit a psychiatric diagnosis as their emotional problems are not severe and should probably be regarded as distress disorders. Between 50 and

70 per cent of patients presenting to primary-care physicians complain solely of pain and conceal emotional disturbance. In comparison with other chronic pain groups, facial pain patients have the lowest rate of psychological illness.

The complaint of facial pain often leads to a specialist referral (Fig. 4.2). The specialists consulted may have neither the time nor the training to discuss emotional problems (Oakley *et al.* 1989). Therefore a number of investigations may be undertaken before a 'functional' diagnosis is made. The investigation and speculative management of these patients utilizes an enormous amount of energy of medical and dental practitioners. Not only do negative investigations cost money, they may also demoralize both patient and doctor.

What is required is some way in which emotional disturbance can be identified before patients are subject to a battery of physical investigations. Early identification of problems may also affect the development and persistence of somatization itself (Katon *et al.* 1990). The reaction of others and, paradoxically, the bland reassurance provided by many doctors that 'nothing serious is wrong' may be a vital factor in causing acute symptoms to become chronic (Kellner 1986).

Childhood experience and health behaviour

The investigation and appropriate management of patients with unexplained medical symptoms requires an understanding of why somatizing patterns develop (Mayou *et al.* 1995). Several investigations have implicated stressful life events in the genesis of facial pain. The main problem with collecting life event data is retrospective reporting. Inaccuracy of recall may be compounded by attempts to explain the

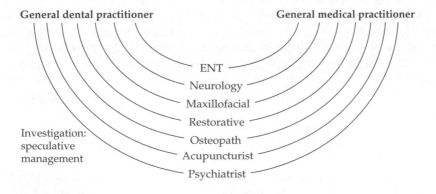

Fig. 4.2 Pathways to care for chronic idiopathic facial pain.

illness in terms of real and imagined stress, or by misperceptions due to depression or demoralization resulting from chronic pain itself.

There is increasing evidence to suggest that unexplained medical symptoms such as orofacial pain affect individuals who have a childhood experience of illness, family ill health, or sexual and physical abuse (Mayou *et al.* 1995). The similarity between the patients' symptoms and those of their parents is particularly striking. Associated lack of care or abuse leads to development of low self-esteem and abnormal health beliefs and behaviour (Barsky *et al.* 1994). Craig *et al.* (1993) also found that the best predictors of adult somatization were parental lack of care and childhood illness. Facial pain patients appear to be psychologically and biochemically vulnerable. The psychosocial features of importance include an unstable or inadequate parental background, poor adaptation to school or work, marital and financial difficulties, chronic illness in the family, and bereavement (Feinmann and Harris 1984*a*; Speculand *et al.* 1984). However, Marbach *et al.* (1988) did not find any difference between patients and controls as far as adverse life events are concerned, but found that patients had fewer sources of emotional support and coped less well. Feinmann and Harris (1984*a*) have shown that 43 per cent of such patients were psychiatrically normal, 35 per cent had a depressive illness, and 22 per cent were diagnosed as mixed neurosis. A small number can be identified as having a personality disorder with marked somatization or frank psychosis. The question is how to explain the nature and relationship of the painful peripheral experience to a central psychological disturbance.

In adult life repeated stresses cause emotional arousal, with persistent symptoms which are then accompanied by dysphoria and other psychiatric problems. This may well affect the interpretation of physical symptoms as being indicative of physical illness, leading to recurrent consultations which then become maintaining factors in the transition from acute somatization to chronic pain (Fig. 4.2).

The medical response to pain problems is crucial, it should be based on a coherent protocol to rationalize investigations and treatment in order to prevent chronic somatization. Mayou *et al.* (1995) have proposed a 'multicausal interactive aetiological model' in which subjective symptoms, both physical and psychological, are the results of the patient's interpretation (or attribution) of somatic perceptions (Fig. 4.1).

Thus there are many variables that make it more likely that individuals will amplify normal bodily sensations. These include the ability to identify illness and previous illness experience, including general satisfaction with doctors and medical care. The rest of this chapter considers the roles of the health professionals involved in patient care.

MANAGEMENT

The role of the dental practitioner

The American Dental Association (Griffiths 1983) concluded that only conservative reversible forms of therapy, including drug treatment such as analgesics or antidepressants, could be recommended. A warm, positive, and reassuring attitude on the part of the clinician was considered crucial. Many forms of physical therapy, including bite guards, exercises, local analgesia or heat, cold sprays, short-wave diathermy, and ultrasound, have their supporters but their action is non-specific and most modalities leave a residuum of unresponsive cases or relapses. The more recent NIH 1996 statement has stressed the need for dentists to practice evidence-based care. The traditional role of the general dental practitioner is to exclude problems and refer to a specialist for help. It is important that the general practitioner does not overinvestigate the patient but carries out an agreed treatment plan and asks for help when in trouble. Chapter 3 includes details on how the dentist should exclude physical problems. The dentist should take the APA advice (Chapter 1) and manage the referral appropriately, so that the patient does not feel abandoned or made to feel that his pain is imaginary.

Dental management

It may be difficult for a dentist within a general practice to identify someone who has atypical facial pain. The clinician should recognize that a long-standing severe pain with no characteristic provoking or relieving factors and no neurological or radiological signs is unlikely to have a local basis.

A patient must not be diagnosed as having this condition without a full assessment being made. This almost always requires a number of visits and diagnostic investigative tests. The basis is a detailed history supplemented by special tests such as pulpal vitality testing and the use of high-quality intraoral radiographs. When making a diagnosis of dental or facial pain, it is always necessary to have two or more signs on which to base the diagnosis. These might be the history coupled with the results of vitality testing, or the history combined with radiographic evidence. Symptoms alone are not enough upon which to proceed.

Pain of periodontal or pulpal origin has some typical characteristics, such as reaction to thermal stimuli, pain on creation or release of pressure, spontaneous pain particularly on going to sleep at night. Furthermore, such pain may radiate from one jaw into another or from the lower teeth to the ear, but will almost absolutely never cross the midline of the face. It is often necessary to remove existing restorations from the teeth in order to confirm the diagnosis. However, without two or more diagnostic signs it is not good practice to remove a pulp from a tooth on the basis that so doing might alleviate the problem. If a dental practitioner is uncertain about the cause of dental pain as diagnostic signs are absent, time should be allowed for the pain to localize or for the symptoms to become more characteristic. Discussion with the patient is clearly important and particularly so when a delay in taking specific action to alleviate pain is being considered.

When a dentist is unsure of the location of pain, the use of local analgesia can be helpful in isolating a tooth or teeth as potential causes; however, it is unreliable in patients affected by atypical facial pain and in this group is not of diagnostic significance.

The most difficult of the special tests is the reaction of teeth to heat. Classically the use of a warmed stick of gutta-percha is recommended; however, this does not produce consistent results in every case. There may be benefit in using hot water, not hot enough to burn the mouth but warm enough to be hot. If the patient holds this in the area under suspicion, this will frequently produce a positive response where warmed gutta-percha will not.

The intraoral radiographs must be of good quality. These are essential for determining the presence or absence of dental caries, the depth of existing restorations, and the status of the periodontal ligament space. Long-cone periapical radiographs of the teeth taken using a paralleling device are necessary: these may be supported by bitewing radiographs, which give a better view of the coronal restorations in the teeth, and by further periapical films taken from a different angle in order to parallax views in the case of suspected root perforations or root fractures. The limitations of two-dimensional images of three-dimensional structures should also be borne in mind.

The use of orthopantomograms for restorative dental diagnosis is to be deprecated. These films, although useful as a dental screen, do not provide sufficient detail for making a diagnosis related to the teeth.

It is also important that the dentist is not too quick in the use of local analgesia when teeth are to be investigated. If loss of vitality of a tooth is suspected, it is prudent either to remove any existing restorations without local analgesia or, if the tooth is sound, to prepare a test cavity. The latter is normally the beginning of an access cavity for root canal treatment.

When a restoration is removed, it is important that a provisional restoration is placed which provides a good coronal seal. This should be of zinc oxide–eugenol, which is better if used in a reinforced formulation. However, it produces a marked inflammatory reaction if placed in direct contact with the pulp. If the cavity is deep and a microexposure of the pulp is possible, a base of hard-setting calcium hydroxide should be placed prior to use of the zinc oxide–eugenol temporary restoration.

The patient should be asked to monitor his own condition for either improvement or deterioration, even if such a change is short-lived. No change at all is indicative that the correct tooth was probably not identified; it is also characteristic of patients who have atypical facial pain, where none of the investigations of the teeth makes matters better or worse. A change in the symptoms following investigation is generally indicative that the tooth responsible for the pain has been treated, although it may be one of a group investigated at one appointment.

If the dentist reaches the stage where the teeth in the area affected by the pain have been investigated reasonably and no abnormality found, atypical facial pain may be suspected. However, it is not a diagnosis to be reached lightly without an accurate history having been taken and a thorough investigation having been carried out.

It bears stating again that pulpal devitalization and other aspects of surgery cannot be justified on grounds of pain alone. Although the literature details that patients with this condition give histories that are atypical, this is not always the case. The joint multidisciplinary clinic run for a number of years by the authors has recorded that a number of patients eventually diagnosed as suffering from atypical facial pain consistently gave histories that were entirely characteristic of pulpal or endodontic disorders. The importance of a detailed history, full use of special diagnostic tests, and substantiated intervention bears re-emphasis.

Dentists, when faced by a patient with long-standing facial pain, must balance two different requirements. The first is the obligation to take a thorough history, to carry out a detailed examination, and, if indicated, to carry out further diagnostic tests and investigations. The second is not to overinvestigate or repeat invasive tests that have been carried out previously by others. This produces a tension in most dentists who have frequently been trained to expect a physical cause for most dental and facial symptoms and can lead to a feeling of not having looked after a patient 'properly' if investigations carried out by others with a negative result are not repeated just to make sure that nothing has been missed. The clinician should recognize that a long-standing severe pain with no characteristic provoking or relieving factors and no neurological or radiological signs is unlikely to have an organic basis.

Unfortunately, many patients manifest a lack of psychological insight and are reluctant to accept an emotional explanation for their pain, but insist that an organic cause must be found. This has considerable clinical importance in that they may decline drug therapy or psychiatric help but will readily submit to surgery. Furthermore, the precise localization by the patient, together with unsubstantiated descriptions of swelling, ulceration, discharge, or haemorrhage often encourage the dentist to intervene surgically.

This can vary from the denervation or extraction of a tooth, the exploration of the antrum, to the excision of the salivary gland or sectioning of a division of the trigeminal or glossopharyngeal nerves. The outcome of such surgery may give relief for a short period, often no more than 10 days, and then the pain returns. Such surgery is invariably justified as an exploratory procedure, but is essentially a failure to recognize the existence of the underlying emotional disturbance and the need for its appropriate therapy. Temporary relief by infiltrating the pain site with local anaesthetic is commonly achieved but has no diagnostic significance.

Box 4.2   The role of the general dental practitioner

1. To exclude dental disease.
2. To use conservative treatment methods.
3. To detect emotional concern.
4. To refer appropriately.

The role of the dental specialist

A crucial aspect of the dental specialist's role is to exclude dental disease as detailed above. The specialist may consider fitting an occlusal splint for a short period; however, there are many concerns about the continued use of physical treatment for the management of pain. The rationale for dentists continuing to provide occlusal appliances for the treatment of temporomandibular dysfunction and the protection of the teeth in bruxism has been discussed previously. However, the provision of such an appliance must produce no irreversible change to the position of the teeth or the relationship between the maxilla and the mandible. The soft vinyl mouthguard type of appliance constructed by vacuum forming on a study cast may be effective in the short term. However, it appears to be less effective than a stabilization appliance made of hard acrylic resin, and although the soft type may be appropriate for initial management in an acute presentation, the latter type may prove to be more effective for longer and it is also available for intermittent use as it is considerably more durable. If the appliance is to be reversible, it must cover all of the functional surfaces of the teeth and must present an occlusal surface free of all indentations so that the mandible is not maintained in any predetermined position on closure. In order to assist dentists in the management of this condition in primary care, the construction of the splint is described in Appendix 1.

Management

It is unfortunate that articles and texts still describe the role of adjustment of the occlusion as a means of controlling temporomandibular dysfunction. Indeed, it has been written relatively recently that those dentists not availing their patients of the benefits of occlusal adjustment in the treatment of this condition were practising dentistry badly. The evidence linking occlusion abnormalities with temporomandibular dysfunction was reviewed carefully by Okeson (1996). On the basis of the current literature, it is impossible to support occlusal equilibration as a treatment modality for the condition.

The role of occlusal appliances in the management of the condition is more equivocal. They are intended to provide one or more of the following: relaxation of the mandibular elevator muscles, protection of the teeth from excessive loads, stabilization of the temporomandibular joint, and to eliminate bruxism. If the condition is truly associated with increased levels of muscle activity, as originally suggested by Ramfjord and Ash (1995), one way of reducing the activity of the masticatory muscles is by increasing the vertical dimension of the patient's occlusion (i.e. by separating the teeth and increasing face height on mandibular closure). This can be achieved readily by provision of an occlusal appliance. Electromyogram (EMG) studies indicate that this results in a decrease in mandibular elevator activity (Okeson 1996; Shan and Yun 1991).

There are numerous designs of appliance and in this area of particular empiricism there is little objective basis upon which to select a particular type. However, certain criteria should be fulfilled. The American Dental Association (Griffiths 1983) recommended that occlusal therapy for TMD should be reversible. Such recommendations can be most readily fulfilled by an appliance that covers all of the teeth in one arch, thereby preventing unwanted changes in the position of the teeth. Doubt has been cast of the reversibility of even these appliances by Wise (personal communication, 1996), who has stated that wear of such an appliance led to a permanent change in the mandibulo-maxillary relationship. However, there are no other reports recording the same happening, and the essentially reversible nature of the treatment afforded by such appliances remains one of their attractions. There has, however, been a significant change in the regimes employed in their use. Adjustment of the natural dentition should generally not be considered, there being no indication that it is either beneficial or even necessary. (Appendix 1 has a detailed description of the construction of an occlusal appliance.)

The patient is provided with an occlusal splint which is adjusted to provide stable, even contacts for the opposing teeth and to facilitate smooth mandibular movements in excursions away from the position of closure. Wearing such an appliance, carefully adjusted, may give symptomatic relief for a short period of time. After a period of wear, the patient is asked to stop using it and only to recommence wear if symptoms return. Such a regime generally proves acceptable. The nature of the condition is such that recurrences are not infrequent. The patient therefore keeps the appliance and is able to start wearing it again if symptoms return. The appliance is seen only as part of the management, which centres on patient explanation, reassurance about the nature and course of the condition, and conservative reversible therapy, of which the occlusal splint may be just one option. The major criticism of this approach lies in the fact that controlled clinical trials are not currently available to substantiate it, while it is not apparent that alternative and even more conservative approaches may yield equally successful results (Turk *et al.* 1993). However, patients with temporomandibular dysfunction continue to present to dental practitioners in the expectation of 'cure' and the apparent usefulness of such treatment is documented (Clark 1984). Dentists have, by and large, been trained to provide oral management for such conditions and may consider themselves insufficiently trained in the long-term monitoring of patients taking medication for this condition. If occlusal appliances are dismissed as being inappropriate, the management of vast numbers of patients within a primary-care setting becomes improbable and the burden on the secondary referral tier would become immense. Under present circumstances there still remains a role for very conservative management, which includes physical therapy in the form of an occlusal appliance which will not produce changes to the position of the teeth or the relationship between the maxilla and mandible. However, the dentist must remain aware of the limitations of such treatment and must consider referring the patient for alternative management if no response to treatment is obtained. The authors, in their joint management of this condition, have recognized that one treatment modality is not necessarily applicable or acceptable to all patients, while it is recognized that to consider a pure occlusal cause for the condition is inappropriate. There appears at present to be merit in considering the recent Scientific Statement from the National Institutes of Health (NIH) (1996). This concluded that treatment for temporomandibular dysfunction should be based on the use of conservative and reversible therapeutic modalities. It further stated that no specific therapies had been shown to be universally or uniformly effective.

However, it concluded that many conservative modalities provided palliative relief while not producing harm (Greene *et al.* 1998).

Physical treatment

Franks (1965) in one of the earliest controlled bite guard trials, achieved 80 per cent improvement after 4 weeks of nocturnal wear. This reflects many similar trials conducted since. However, on closer scrutiny of these results only 20 per cent were 'cured' (i.e. pain free). Green and Laskin (1972) have also shown that 40 per cent of patients improve with a placebo bite guard. Feinmann and Harris (1984*b*) found that compliance with a soft lower bite guard rapidly diminished so that only a third of patients wore one after 9 weeks of therapy. Recent clinical studies frequently combine the use of intraoral appliances with other modes of therapy, creating difficulty in the interpretation of results. Short-term efficacy of splint therapy alone was indicated in recent well-designed studies by Turk *et al.* (1993). In the latter study at 5–7 weeks, treatment with an intraoral appliance worn 24 hours a day was significantly more effective in reducing pain intensity than a placebo palatal splint worn 24 hours a day or an intraoral appliance worn 30 minutes a day. However, at 10 weeks all treatments were equally effective. This may therefore reflect poor compliance or decreased efficacy of the appliance after 7 weeks.

The most frequently constructed appliances, currently used in the treatment of temporomandibular joint (TMJ) problems, are the flat-plane stabilization appliances and the full-arch anterior repositioning appliances (Okeson 1996). Complications may arise with the use of any appliance when used incorrectly or worn excessively. Problems include caries, periodontal involvement, psychological dependence, or, in some cases, uncontrolled occlusal alteration, as indicated by Abbott and Bush (1991).

Evidence-based splint therapy

Raphael and Marbach (1997) have summarized the need for evidence-based care of musculoskeletal facial pain. This work is based on the National Institutes of Health Technology assessment on the management of TMJ (NIH 1996). The conference noted that dental practitioners relied on clinical observation rather than evaluating treatment efficacy. The authors have conducted a Cochrane-style review of the efficacy of splint therapy and draw readers' attention to factors that can lead to incorrect conclusions about treatment efficacy when relying on clinical observation. These are:

- placebo effects of treatment;
- regression to the mean;
- spontaneous remission;
- natural variability of signs and symptoms;
- failure to consider treatment dropouts;
- bias in self-reports of symptom remission.

Statistical regression occurs when extreme scores that are invariably measured inaccurately (pain symptom severity) move closer to the mean level when measurement is repeated. Raphael and Marbach critically reviewed the literature concerned with the usefulness of intraoral appliances, and concluded that despite their widespread use in clinical practice the best design research studies do not support the user of intraoral appliances. Indeed, the NIH committee concluded that the preponderance of data does not support the superiority of any method for initial management of most temporomandibular dysfunction (TMD) problems. The superiority of such methods to placebo controls or no treatment controls remains undetermined. The dentist must therefore exclude disease and attempt symptomatic management and then refer appropriately.

Medical management: liaison psychiatry

Once dental pathology is excluded or judged to be not of primary importance, the next step is the involvement of a specialist psychiatric or psychological service, and it must be emphasized that this is best provided within a dental setting. The manner of referral to the specialist is of great significance as the patient must not feel abandoned. Joint management by dental specialist and psychiatrist may be appropriate. Certainly discussion is important, in some cases the general dental practitioner (GDP) will only be seeking reassurance that his long-term treatment is correct. Liaison psychiatry in the United Kingdom is a relatively scarce resource. Less than half the districts surveyed recently had a designated consultant psychiatrist with overall responsibility for general hospital service, and fewer had a full liaison psychiatry team. This is in sharp contrast to some other European countries that have a liaison psychiatry service in each district hospital (Mayou *et al.* 1990). The shortage and need for improved liaison psychiatry in the United Kingdom has been emphasized in a recent joint report of the Royal College of Physicians and Psychiatrists (Royal College of Physicians 1989). Also, there are few pain clinics in the United Kingdom that have had the experience of working with liaison psychiatry.

A specialist clinic which assesses the patient may be in oral medicine, maxillofacial surgery, conservation or liaison psychiatry. It must be

---

Box 4.3 The role of the dental specialist

1. To exclude treatable disease. Persistence of symptoms in the face of conservative treatment requires referral to a dental specialist, who will have access to further diagnostic tests and who will be in a position to review previous treatment. The basis for continued investigation is a careful and full history both of the course and symptoms of the condition and the outcome of previous treatment. The general dental practitioner is well placed to assist the specialist by providing available dental records, including radiographs. These may help in characterizing the problem and prevent repeated investigation.

2. To give a clear message about the absence of disease. The patient must be aware of the diagnosis and the presence and absence of disease. Further investigations may be necessary to exclude dental and orofacial disease. The specialist must stress the absence of pathology, when none is revealed, as continued investigation and treatment reinforce the patient's perception that he must have a dental problem. The great challenge for the specialist is to be thorough and diligent in diagnosis and management without following a course of overinvestigation.

3. To co-ordinate management and refer appropriately. The dental specialist is well placed to co-ordinate management. He can provide confirmation that a dental cause for the problem is unlikely and provide the patient with sufficient information to enable making a joint and informed decision about future management.

---

remembered that some hospital colleagues and departments may be more psychologically minded than others, and such sympathies will determine the situation of the clinic. It is important to try to refer at an early stage, rather than when it is decided that there 'is nothing wrong' with the patient, refer to a psychiatrist. Wherever the patient is seen, adequate assessment is crucial. Why did this patient become ill? It is essential to make it clear that the patient's symptoms are real. All complaints must be taken seriously and should proceed in a sequence from the physical symptoms to psychological topics (see p. 109). A history will inevitably include discussion of previous treatments, but also family and past medical history and attitudes to illness in the patient's upbringing. Assessment may take more than one interview, and should include an assessment of mood. It may be helpful to use a rating scale to quantify physical and psychological symptoms (see Chapter 1).

Box 4.4   Assessment
- Why is the patient here?
- Assess complaints.
- Review previous treatments.
- Review family history.
- Assess childhood experience.
- Assess mood.

The treatment offered will depend on the diagnosis and available clinical resources. Compliance is better if there is a shared understanding of illness. Helping the patient be aware of tension and to identify sources of stress is important. The workplace may be a cause of stress and negotiations with employers may be important. Many patients have maladaptive coping strategies, such as avoidance of personal conflicts and lack of assertiveness, and may be helped by simple advice about these issues. Others will benefit from advice about relaxation and breathing control. The main goal of cognitive behavioural therapy (CBT) is to get the patient to take control of his problems, and self-help is, in effect, a way of achieving this (see Chapter 6). It is crucial that the practitioner sees self-help as an ally. Lack of sympathy or a patronizing attitude to the treatment may drive the patient away.

Drug therapy

For the majority of patients, particularly those seen in primary care, informed reassurance is sufficient. When drug treatment is prescribed, antidepressants should be taken at night in slowly increasing doses, combined with regular review at intervals of 3–6 weeks to provide re-assurance and achieve compliance. Sedation is rarely required, so a tricyclic antidepressant with low sedative and low anticholingergic side-effects, such as nortriptyline, is recommended. Nortriptyline (Allegron®) may be increased gradually from 10 to 30 mg/day, and then from 50 to 100 mg/day. The selective serotonin reuptake inhibitors such as fluoxetine (Prozac®), offer a useful alternative, if tolerated in dosages of 20–60 mg daily, taken in the morning to prevent insomnia.

The particular advantages of the SSRIs are: no weight gain, no sedation or xerostomia, and no interference with driving, The efficacy of fluoxetine has been demonstrated in a recent study (Harrison *et al.* 1997).

Two new agents, venlafaxine (Efexor®) 37.5 mg daily and nefazodone (Dutonin®) 100–200 mg twice daily, inhibit the reuptake of noradrenaline and serotonin; and reboxetine (Edronax®) 4–8 mg daily and mirtazapine (Zispin®) 15–45 mg inhibit noradrenaline and dopamine, have fewer side-effects and are safer in overdose than TCAs, but their efficacy in pain control is not yet proven.

For those patients with insomnia, a sedating tricyclic such as dothiepin is useful, starting with a single night-time dose of 25 mg and increasing in steps up to 225 mg at night where necessary. In elderly patients with constipation or glaucoma, and in males with prostatic hypertrophy, the least anticholinergic drug should be prescribed. It must be remembered that individuals react to different drugs in different ways and the clinician must be flexible in prescribing.

Palpitations from an anxious state or from the antidepressant drug therapy can be controlled with a β-blocker such as propranolol (40 mg two or three times a day). β-Blockers also have a useful effect in their own right on idiopathic face and head pains. Medication should be continued for at least 3–6 months, and for years in some cases. It should always be withdrawn slowly and any relapse of pain indicates the need for a reintroduction of medication. Some patients need strong encouragement and clear directives to enhance compliance. This is facilitated by a 'handout' which explains that the drugs have a non-psychotropic pain control action which may involve a direct effect on the blood vessels as well as a central analgesic action (see Appendices 2 and 3). The fact that tricyclic antidepressants are used to treat migraine, arthritis, post-herpetic neuralgia, diabetic neuropathy, terminal pain, and other chronic pains should also be stressed. Side-effects that include dry mouth, drowsiness, palpitations, constipation, and urinary hesitancy are not common and rarely severe.

Furthermore, when warned of these, some patients are unfortunately subject to 'placebo side-effects' which have been shown to exceed those of the active drug (Feinmann and Harris 1984*b*). The side-effects of the SSRIs generally disappear after a few weeks but some patients may have persistent headaches, nausea, insomnia, and sexual problems.

Which antidepressant?

The choice of which antidepressant to use is dependent on adverse effects, interactions, and overdose. The unwanted effects may vary from mild and tolerable to potentially lethal. In addition to the original two main groups of antidepressants—the tricyclic antidepressants (TCAs) and the monoamine oxidase inhibitors (MAOIs)—recent years have seen the introduction of a number of newer drugs, with a wide range of chemical structures and differing pharmacological activities. They also

Table 4.5 More common adverse effects of different antidepressant drugs compared

Drug	Anticholinergic effect	Sedation	Stimulant effect	Nausea	Convulsant effect	Cardiac effects	Toxicity in overdose
Tricyclic antidepressants							
Amitriptyline	+++	+++	0	+	++	+++	+++
Amoxapine	+++	+	0	0	+++	+	+++
Clomipramine	++	+	0	+	++	++	++
Desipramine	+	+	0	+	+	++	++
Dothiepin	++	++	0	0	++	++	+++
Doxepin	++	++	0	0	++	++	++
Imipramine	+++	++	0	+	++	++	+++
Lofepramine	+	+	0	0	0	+	0
Nortriptyline	++	++	0	+	+	++	++
Protriptyline	++	+	0	+	+	+	+++
Trimipramine	+++	++	0	0	+	++	++
Monoamine oxidase inhibitors (MAO)							
Iproniazid	0	0	++	+	0	0	++
Isocarboxazid	0	0	+	++	0	+	+++
Phenelzine	0	0	+	+	0	0	++
Tranylcypromine	0	0	+++	+	0	0	++

Reversible inhibitors of monoamine oxidase A (RIMA)

Moclobemide	0	0	+	+	0	0	+

Selective serotonin reuptake inhibitors (SSRIs)

Citalopram	0	0	++	0	0	+	+
Fluvoxamine	0	+	+++	0	+	+	0
Fluoxetine	0	+	0	++	0	0	0
Sertraline	0	0	++	0	0	0	0

Atypical drugs

Maprotiline	++	++	+	0	+++	++	+++
Mianserin	0	+++	0	0	0	0	0
Nefazodone	0	0	++	0	0	0	I
Trazodone	0	++	+++	0	0	+	+
Venlafaxine	0	0	++	0	I	0	I
Viloxazine	+	+	++	0	0	0	0

Safety of administration in patients with heart problems (angina, arrhythmias, etc.).
+++, very strong; ++, strong; +, mild or absent; I, insufficient information.
Table reproduced by kind permission of the Royal College of Psychiatrists.

have a new spectrum of adverse effects and interactions. The most important limitations of TCAs are prostatic obstruction, narrow-angle glaucoma, and some cardiac conditions.

Most of the TCAs are contraindicated within 3 months of a myocardial infarction or in patients under treatment for heart failure. These drugs are also more likely to cause postural hypotension in the elderly. However, the newer drugs also produce adverse effects, which may limit their use in certain circumstances (Table 4.5). Lofepramine can be considered a newer tricyclic drug and has milder anticholergic effects than the other TCAs. The most common adverse effects caused by the different antidepressants are compared in Table 4.6. Other toxic effects are uncommon.

Rashes occur with most drugs, including fluoxetine, and liver damage can occur with the TCAs and lofepramine. The anticholinergic effects of TCAs can be diminished by starting at a lower than therapeutic dose. Tolerance soon occurs to the nausea caused by the selective serotonin

Table 4.6   Adverse effects of antidepressants

Tricyclics

Dry mouth, blurred vision, constipation, urinary retention, drowsiness, postural hypotension

Moclobemide

Insomnia, dizziness, nausea, headache, restlessness, agitation, confusion

Monoamine oxidase inhibitors

Dry mouth, blurred vision, constipation, urinary retention, drowsiness (sometimes insomnia), tremor, dizziness, weakness, fatigue, gastrointestinal

Selective serotonin reuptake inhibitors

Citalopram: nausea, sweating, tremor, drowsiness, dry mouth
Fluoxetine: nausea, headache, nervousness, insomnia, anxiety, dizziness, weakness
Fluvoxamine: nausea, vomiting, drowsiness, diarrhoea, agitation, tremor, hypokinesia, asthenia
Paroxetine: constipation, insomnia, dry mouth, tremor, weakness, sweating, nausea, drowsiness, headache
Sertraline: dry mouth, nausea, diarrhoea, tremor, sweating, dyspepsia, ejaculatory delay

Nefazodone

Weakness, dry mouth, nausea, dizziness, drowsiness

Venlafaxine

Nausea, headache, drowsiness, insomnia, dry mouth, dizziness, constipation, weakness, nervousness reuptake inhibitors (SSRIs). Attrition due to side-effects is 10 per cent lower with SSRI treatment than during treatment with TCAs.

Interactions

The 'cheese' interaction with the older MAOIs is very well known, and consists of a hypertensive crisis provoked by certain food and drugs. This interaction is much less likely to occur with the new selective inhibitors of monoamine oxidase, such as moclobemide, and restriction of diet is not required provided the patient does not indulge in binges of contraindicated foods. Some of the SSRIs, especially fluoxetine, may increase the adverse effects of lithium, and although the TCAs are normally well tolerated with lithium, there may rarely be myoclonus and seizures.

Since many of the newer drugs are serotoninergic, the possibility of provoking a serotonin syndrome by simultaneously prescribing drugs with a serotoninergic mode of action (the five SSRIs, clomipramine, nefazodone, and venlafaxine) needs to be considered carefully. In most cases this involves introducing the drug gradually by titrating the dose upwards and telling the patient not to take any further doses if they experience any untoward symptoms. The syndrome presents as progressive restlessness, hyper-reflexia, shivering, tremor, and sweating, due to an excess of serotonin at a synaptic level. Agitation, confusion, and hypomanic behaviour may occur. The pupils are usually widely dilated. If muscle spasms are severe, or if the patient develops a pyrexia, urgent medical attention will be required. Drugs such as propranolol or cypropheptadine may be used for their antiserotoninergic effect. In extreme cases, paralysis with muscle relaxants and mechanical ventilation may be required. Since the syndrome includes muscle stiffness and rigidity, restlessness, agitation, and a raised temperature, it needs to be considered in the differential diagnosis of neuroleptic malignant syndrome.

Nemeroff *et al.* (1996) warn that drug interactions may occur in patients treated with combinations of drugs that inhibit a particular P450 enzyme. Three SSRIs—paroxetine, fluoxetine, and sertraline—increase plasma concentrations of drugs metabolized by P450, including the tricylic antidepressants. The newer drugs, venlafaxine and mirtazapine, appear not to inhibit any of these enzymes and are therefore less likely to cause interactions.

Another type of interaction which must be taken in to account is the oxidative enzyme inhibiting properties of the SSRIs. Several of these drugs have the capacity to inhibit the hepatic metabolism of drugs that the patient may be receiving. The plasma level of some TCAs may be raised by this mechanism. SSRIs such as fluvoxamine and setraline can prolong the prothrombin time by inhibiting the metabolism of warfarin.

Paroxetine also prolongs prothrombin time, but in addition may further increase the tendency to bleeding; the reason for this is not fully established. Therefore this drug should be used with extreme caution in any patient on warfarin.

Changing between antidepressants

Quite frequently the antidepressant first chosen does not produce the desired effect, and treatment needs to be changed to another drug. When introducing a new drug, the question of antidepressant–antidepressant interactions must be considered. The problem is compounded by the long elimination half-lives of some antidepressants, particularly fluoxetine, and the time taken for the pharmacological effect to disappear, which is particularly notable in the case of the older MAOIs. One exception is moclobemide, which in most cases requires no treatment-free interval when introducing a new drug, because its persistence in the body is short. Thus the time factor deserves close consideration, particularly when changing antidepressants, especially with drugs such as fluoxetine, which has a long persistence in the body (up to 35 days; a 7-day interval is usually sufficient for other SSRIs, trazodone, nefazodone, and venlafaxine), and the older MAOIs (interactions may occur up to 14 days after discontinuation).

Additional strategies

In intractable cases, first cognitive therapy (Harrison *et al.* 1997) or hypnotherapy more intensive psychotherapy (Guthrie 1996) should be considered. Hahn *et al.* (1994) suggest that health professionals should examine the doctor–patient interaction to include that relationship in strategies for managing the difficult patient. It may be that a defensive attitude on the practitioner's behalf prevents the patient achieving pain relief.

Duration of treatment

All patients should remain on medication for at least 3 months and, in some cases, up to a year to prevent further relapse. Reviewing the long-term prognosis of pain, Feinmann (1993) found that between 60 and 70 per cent of patients are pain free at 4-year follow-up, but about 50 per cent of patients experienced short-term return of symptoms in association with stress. Forty per cent of the patients had to be maintained on medication for 1 year to prevent relapse and 20 per cent were still taking medication at 4 years. Freedom from pain at 12 months was associated with an adverse life event, such as bereavement, prior to the pain developing, implying that counselling of identifiable causes has a good prognosis (Table 4.7). An early response to drug treatment was also a strong predictor of freedom from pain after 1 year. If there was no improvement after 2 months of therapy, the pain was unchanged at 12 months. Patients who remained in pain were characterized by a long history of ill health as well as previous unsuccessful dental and surgical treatment for pain. Patients who remained in pain at 4 years were preoccupied by pain and had 'neuroticism scores' which were higher than their original scores, indicating that complaining behaviour is reflected by these scores.

As some patients have to be maintained on medication for at least a year to prevent relapse, psychogenic facial pain and headache should be considered to be a chronic recurrent disturbance such as migraine or trigeminal neuralgia and treated with a comparable continuous medical regime.

The majority of patients can be discharged to primary care, but a small group will require long-term follow-up in specialist clinics to prevent excessive investigation elsewhere (Fig. 4.3).

Lipton and Marbach (1984), in a long-term follow-up study, showed that the patient's socio-cultural background, treatment history, and response and attitude to pain were more important than clinical signs in predicting pain relief. Orbach and Dworkin (1998) examined 235 cases at 5-year follow-up: 49 per cent remitted, 14 per cent improved, 9 per cent showed low improvement, 13 per cent were the same, and 16 per cent were worse. The 5-year outcome in pain was largely independent of changes in clinical signs and dependent on psychosocial problems. This suggests that the separation of the various facial pain symptoms into different diagnostic groups is less important than previously thought. Patients should be assessed in terms of their psychological problems and understanding of pain. The failure to recognize the importance of patients' emotional problems has, in the past, led to an excess of physical treatment which, unfortunately, has caused an increase in complaints about treatment. Litigation arises from a lack of agreement between

Table 4.7 Past history of patients pain free and in pain at 12 months

	Pain free ($n = 68$)	In pain ($n = 16$)
Frequent ill health	6 (9%)	5 (31%)*
Unsuccessful surgical treatment	22 (32%)	15 (94%)*
Life event prior to pain development	43 (63%)	1 (6%)*

* $P < 0.05$.

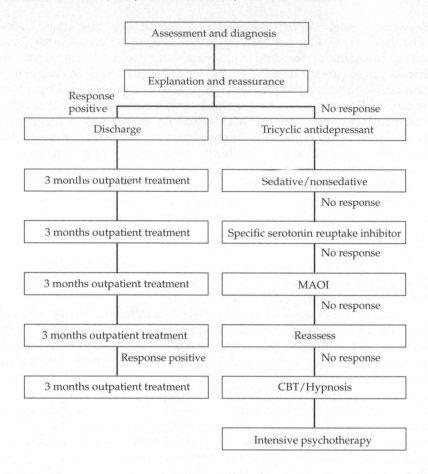

Fig. 4.3 Clinical algorithm of facial pain.

patients and dentists and doctors as to the cause of pain and appropriate treatment.

Antidepressant drugs are universally available and cheap. They are often the treatment of first choice for facial pain patients, instead of psychological treatment which is more expensive and in short supply. There is reasonable evidence for their efficacy in chronic facial pain.

Lascelles (1966) showed that phenelzine (Nardil®) was effective in atypical facial pain and since then a variety of the less troublesome tricyclic antidepressants (TCAs) have been used in FAM and related pain problems, such as tension headaches and severe recurrent migraine.

In a double-blind controlled trial (Feinmann and Harris 1984b) the tricyclic antidepressant drug dothiepin (Prothiaden®) was found to be superior to placebo in the relief of facial pain. Seventy-one per cent of dothiepin patients were pain-free at the end of 9 weeks' treatment, compared to 46 per cent of those receiving a placebo.

The observation that nearly half the patients responded to reassurance and a placebo explains why so many diverse forms of treatment appear to be successful. Pain relief was found to be independent of any antidepressant effect of the medication, suggesting that the drug had a central analgesic action appropriate to this form of pain disorder (Feinmann 1985).

In some patients, pain recurrence was associated with withdrawal from medication and the tricyclic antidepressant had to be maintained for at least a year to prevent relapse. In other words, facial pain should be considered to be a chronic recurrent disturbance in the same way as migraine or trigeminal neuralgia, and be treated, when appropriate, by a comparable continuous medical regime.

Onghena and Van Houdenhove (1992) conducted a meta-analysis of 39 placebo-controlled studies in chronic non-malignant pain, and showed the mean size of the analgesic effect to be 0.64—a 74 per cent reduction of pain in the antidepressant-treated group compared to the placebo group. Jung *et al.* (1997), in a review of published data, found that selective serotonin reuptake inhibitors (SSRIs), particularly fluoxetine, were effective for mixed chronic pain. Harrison *et al.* (1997), in a study comparing fluoxetine with cognitive behaviour therapy, has demonstrated the efficacy of fluoxetine in relieving facial pain. The analgesic effect of antidepressants in orofacial pain is now recognized by the *British National Formulary* (BNF 1998). A biochemical basis for chronic facial pain is suggested by the association with depression and the response to tricyclic antidepressants. Magni (1987) has also found a high percentage of emotional disorder in first-degree relatives of chronic pain patients. However, the relief of pain by tricyclic antidepressants occurs just as effectively in non-depressed psychiatrically normal patients.

There are acknowledged difficulties in the management of these patients. The first is to convince some patients that they merely require

---

Box 4.5   Antidepressant pain relief
- Quick; worth trying in most patients.
- Achieved at low doses; independent of depression.
- Some need long-term help.

reassurance and medication as opposed to surgery. Also, many dental specialists are unused to taking a full medical history and are timid about using psychotropic medication, particularly where clinical stamina is required to achieve relief of symptoms in a difficult case.

For this reason a liaison psychiatrist is required with an interest in psychosomatic medicine for unresponsive or emotionally disturbed patients. Patients with clinical and radiographic evidence of secondary changes such as osteoarthritis, meniscus displacement, and even perforation may also respond well to tricyclic drug therapy and become symptom-free. Those with marked inflammatory or degenerative changes should also be given a non-steroidal anti-inflammatory analgesic (NSAID), such as ibuprofen 400–600 mg three times a day with meals, unless the patient has a history of peptic ulceration.

Box 4.6   The role of the specialist psychiatry service

- To provide a service for patients — life-style change, relaxation, drugs.
- To advise other doctors/dentists — drug treatments, support.
- To optimize self-help.

Who should treat

Individual clinicians must decide whether they have the appropriate training and skills to treat orofacial patients. If unsure, they should seek advice or refer the patient to a specialist in oral medicine, maxillofacial surgery, or liaison psychiatry. It may be appropriate for general practitioners to get extra training to help such patients.

It is essential to explain the nature of the condition to the patient as well as providing active therapy. It should be emphasized that the pain is real and not imaginary, arising from cramped muscles and dilated blood vessels as a response to stress. With atypical odontalgia, it is helpful to describe it to the patient as being a migraine variant experienced in the teeth. The patient should be reassured that this is a common problem and that no serious physical or progressive disorder is present. A printed handout is invaluable for communication and reassurance.

Informed reassurance and occasional analgesia with NSAIDs or paracetamol (acetaminophen) is sufficient in some patients. Only essential dentistry should be carried out. The American Dental Association has advocated only reversible therapy, and stressed that the most important aspect of treatment includes a warm, positive, and reassuring attitude on behalf of the clinician (Griffiths 1983). If the patients do not respond to reassurance, or have had previous ineffective therapy, antidepressants should be prescribed.

There are several models of liaison psychiatric services but a joint clinic providing a multidisciplinary assessment model offers a number of advantages. Joint assessment promotes communication and under-standing between different disciplines, particularly with regard to the strengths and limitations of available treatments. Inevitably there is some degree of learning and sharing of skills, but more importantly joint clinics prevent splitting whereby a patient may play one doctor off against another. Of course, not every patient needs to be seen at a joint clinic, but pain clinicians will have a feel for which of their patients are going to be hard to manage and these may be selected out for assessment at joint clinics. A liaison psychiatrist may also need some additional time to follow up these patients on an individual basis, who can then be reassessed as needed in the joint clinic. Patients who are already under psychiatric or psychological care, as frequently occurs in certain medical conditions, will benefit from a co-ordinated approach. If contemplating referring such a patient to a pain management pro-gramme, it is important to liaise with their current therapist or psychiatrist to ensure that conflicting therapies are not employed simultaneously.

Because of current funding arrangements with the NHS internal market, pain clinics will need to arrange their own funding of liaison psychiatry sessions, through persuading the purchaser and attracting the patients from fundholding general practices and then purchasing sessions from the department of psychiatry. This needs to be done with the support of local psychiatrists who may need to accept referrals if things go wrong.

Counselling and changing the agenda

Antidepressants should not be used in isolation. A pragmatic treatment approach must be adopted in which the diagnosis is first established by a careful history which identifies other idiopathic pains and seeks out stressful life events. Many patients will respond to reattribution or 'change of agenda' of their physical symptoms to an emotional cause by an explanation of amplifying normal bodily sensations (Bridges and Goldberg 1985).

Gaske and O'Dowde (1989) have shown that this reattribution model can be successfully taught to GMPs, suggesting that GDPs would also benefit. Hypnosis and relaxation are both helpful. There is also evidence that cognitive behavioural therapy can be effective alone or may

---

Box 4.7   Reattribution, the clinician must:

- Take a full history of the symptoms.
- Explore emotional clues.
- Explore social and family factors.
- Explore health belief.
- Perform a focused physical examination.

Box 4.8   Reattribution, the patient must:

- Feel understood.
- Change focus of attention.
- Make a link between emotional cause and pain.

---

augment and prolong the effect of antidepressant medication (Harrison *et al.* 1997) (see Chapter 6). Group therapy with relaxation techniques may also be helpful (Harrison *et al.* 1997). The patient should also be reassured and counselled in terms of appropriate life style.

Summary of management

A clinical service in which the patient can have confidence is essential. The patients must not feel as though they have reached a dead end in treatment. A sympathetic, caring team must provide an environment in which patients can discuss fears and concerns.

For successful management the following points are important:

1.   To identify not only the features of the joint pain but also chronic pain disorders elsewhere, for example, the head, neck, back, abdomen, and pelvis.

2.   To identify predisposing adverse life events or a history of an emotional or psychiatric disturbance.

3.   To emphasize to the patient that the pain is real rather than imaginary, arising in 'cramped' muscles and dilated blood vessels as a response

to emotional stress, and that drug therapy is not being used to treat depression but has a direct effect in relieving the painful muscles and blood vessels.

4.   To prescribe antidepressants for pain. Tricyclic antidepressant (TCAs) drugs such as nortriptyline 10–100 mg, or selective serotonin reuptake inhibitors (SSRIs) such as fluoxetine 20 mg daily, venlafaxine 37.5 mg twice a day, or nefazodone 100 mg twice a day should be prescribed in gradually increasing doses, combined with regular reviews at 3–6-weekly intervals to provide reassurance and to achieve drug compliance. Little or no response after 12 weeks indicates a need for further investigation and/or additional medication. Reluctance to take medication and placebo side-effects are common problems which are usually overcome with firm reassurance. The majority of patients respond well to these regimes but some will require a psychiatrist to provide diagnostic and therapeutic support. A trial of cognitive therapy versus drug therapy has shown the value of the two treatments alone and together.

5.   A handout is invaluable to aid compliance (Appendix 2). Patients forget explanations as soon as they leave the consulting room. A handout for general medical practitioners (GMPs) and general dental practitioners (GDPs) also assists with management in primary care and avoids a build-up of follow-up patients in specialist clinics (Appendix 3).

6.   Dental treatment should be confined to essential problems such as sensitive carious cavities, pulpal inflammation, or marked occlusal disturbances, usually where there is a gross deficiency of functional teeth. Dental procedures intended to perfect the natural occlusion can create intractable somatopsychic problems which not only obscure the primary aetiology but also complicate treatment. An occlusal appliance worn either at night or during the day between meals to discourage bruxism is used by many clinicians to relive the pain and trismus. It is said to protect the mandibular joint surfaces from excessive compression and inhibit maximal elevator muscle contraction. It may also be the only form of treatment some patients will accept, if they are reluctant either to acknowledge an emotional cause or to take psychotropic drugs even when described as muscle relaxants. However, compliance is unpredictable (for practical advice see Appendix 1).

7.   Only when conservative treatments have been exhausted should an alternative arthroscopic or surgical opinion be sought, although surgery is rarely indicated.

8.   Intractable patients should be reassessed by a consultant and intensive psychological treatment considered (Guthrie 1996).

FACIAL PAIN AND THE LAW

There are two very different ways in which patients with persistent facial pain may become involved in litigation.

Idiopathic facial and temporomandibular joint pain have been associated with physical assault and whiplash injury (Shepherd 1997) and can therefore be a feature of a patient's case for compensation for such injuries. However, on reviewing 34 long-standing cases of facial arthromyalgia, it was noted that the five 'whiplash patients' had the features of post-traumatic stress disorder.

Post-traumatic stress disorder, or PTSD (Agabehgi *et al.* 1992), consists of recurrent 'reliving' of the traumatic event, avoidance of circumstances associated with the trauma, a numbing of general responsiveness, and symptoms of increased arousal, such as insomnia, irritability, or difficulty in concentrating. Psychogenic pain is also a feature of this condition; hence, persistent pain following a stressful injury could well be part of PTSD rather than due to a purely physical internal derangement.

This diagnostic dilemma, not surprisingly, also applies to the whiplash injury itself. Post-traumatic patients involved in compensation litigation appear to suffer more pain than patients who are not to receive pain-contingent benefits. However, they also show marked anxiety and depression and continue to experience significant pain after the settlement of their claims, unless specific care is taken to prevent chronic occurrence. Therefore it is impossible to separate the clinical from the medico-legal management of such cases. The history must not only establish the details of the injury and its temporal relationship to the onset of both pain and dysfunction, it should assess the features of PTSD. This may be aided by use of the event scale questionnaire, as suggested by Horowitz *et al.* (1979) or by referral to a liaison psychiatrist.

Unfortunately, legal action by a patient with chronic pain may be brought against the clinician. The risk is more easily appreciated when considering an audit of 731 new idiopathic facial pain patients seen over 17 months in a department of maxillofacial surgery, which revealed the average duration of pain suffered on referral as being 4.14 years. The median period was 1–2 years (116 patients), and the average number of previous specialist referrals was two.

These data reveal how unsatisfactory facial pain management is, with a substantial number of patients seeking relief for long-standing symptoms. There are at least two recognizable medico-legal presentations. First is the patient with atypical odontalgia for which a conventional dental diagnosis was made. The pain often arises spontaneously, but may also follow a dental procedure, such as a local anaesthetic injection, the fitting of a bridge, or an extraction. Well-intentioned dental therapy to eliminate pain invariably consists of further restorations, root canal therapy, apical surgery, and a course of antibiotics and analgesics. An early diagnosis of chronic psychogenic facial and dental pain and the replacement of dental treatment by medication would prevent the patient from ultimately assuming that his continued suffering implies negligence, for which legal redress is sought.

The second group of patients has a discernible psychiatric illness. This is usually a dysmorphic disorder. In such cases, the patient is obsessive in his conviction that the persistent pain or occlusal discomfort was due entirely to some simple traumatic event or previous professional negligence and that it can be remedied only by the dental treatment that the patient recommends. Unfortunately, the unwitting provision of this treatment not only fails to achieve relief of symptoms, it is rewarded with unpaid fees and long abusive letters to the practitioner or hospital manager, and even to government representatives.

Although such patients see a variety of clinicians, a written psychiatric diagnosis is rarely committed to their voluminous case notes. This reflects reticence on the part of dental specialists to acknowledge the need to identify orofacial psychopathology and to arrange appropriate treatment. Unfortunately, the fear of litigation by all concerned leads to palliative therapy or 'offloading', and eventually a withdrawal of professional help from the patient. Early recognition and a psychiatric diagnosis is essential, together with antipsychotic drug therapy, rather than continued physical or surgical therapy.

With courage and tenacity, it is possible to help most of these intimidating patients. Inappropriate treatment of these conditions has proved a fertile source of litigation, which is showing signs of growth in the UK. Hence the clinician should be aware that liability for both dental and medical negligence is currently governed by the Bolam test—so called from the case of that name in which the following test was propounded: 'A doctor (or dentist) is not negligent if he is acting in accordance with a practice (accepted as proper by a responsible body of medical men skilled in that particular art), merely because there is a body of opinion that takes a contrary view. At the same time, that does not mean that a clinician can obstinately persist with some traditional technique if it has been proved to be contrary to what is really substantially the whole of informed medical opinion'.

A practitioner forced to defend his conduct in the UK would need to be able to call upon suitably experienced consultants who would approve that conduct, and justify that approval by reference to the literature on the topic. However, it is important to realize that with increasing knowledge in any field, that the literature will change, and so should patient management. This raises several important questions for the clinician:

1. Can you establish that you were competent to diagnose and treat the condition? Can you recall the relevant training that you have undergone, and your subsequent reading of relevant articles and textbooks?

2. Can you show that you have taken a proper history and carried out a proper examination? Are your notes sufficiently comprehensive to enable you to recollect what you found and did not find?

3. Are you able to justify your diagnosis and differentiate it from other conditions?

4. Having made your diagnosis, can you show that you were aware of the risks of proceeding with therapy, especially if the patient expressed a reluctance to undergo the treatment, or had a history of an emotional disturbance that would impair a sympathetic relationship between the two of you?

5. Can you show that it was proper for you to treat, rather than to refer?

6. Can you show that you monitored the effects of the treatment, and reconsidered the appropriateness of your treatment if it was proving less than successful?

Obviously for protection against claims for negligence, the practitioner needs to be in a position not only to say that correct treatment has been administered, but to prove it by reference to notes.

Finally, in case these points seem disconcerting, it is the experience of those involved in litigation that patients, at least in the UK, are reluctant to sue practitioners whom they like and who they perceive to have done their best for them. Therefore the cultivation of a sympathetic manner will not only assist treatment, it will provide protection as well.

Conversely, there is anecdotal evidence to suggest that many claimants sue more from a sense of grievance at the failure of the practitioner to apologize or express concern where treatment has failed, than out of a desire for profit. While there is some risk than an apology might be taken as an admission of guilt and be used to begin a claim, on balance it appears that a sincere expression of regret is more likely to prevent claims than to produce them.

IMPROVEMENT OF THE CLINICAL MANAGEMENT OF IDIOPATHIC OROFACIAL PAIN

1. The establishment of multidisciplinary facial pain clinics in dental hospitals and departments of oral and maxillofacial surgery and oral

medicine is desirable. Such groups should minimally comprise an oral physician or maxillofacial surgeon, a liaison psychiatrist, a clinical psychologist, and a nurse specialist. Furthermore, a network of such groups would facilitate clinical research and patient management.

2. Specific training programmes need to be established for medical and dental undergraduates, and medical and dental general practitioners. Although the identification of chronic pain patients may be carried out at both primary- and secondary-care levels, multidisciplinary training programmes will provide a more efficient and cost-effective means of supporting primary care. It will also stop the increasing numbers of patients who resort to litigation when no consensus diagnosis is reached and treatment is unsatisfactory.

3. At present, a disease classification system is premature and may be misleading and inaccurate given (1) the lack of epidemiological information and (2) the identification of as yet undefined aetiologies that are likely to compose the syndrome called facial pain. Carefully designed, analytical, cross-sectional, population-based studies with appropriate clinical measures and biological markers should be conducted to identify the prevalence of presenting signs and symptoms for facial pain, excluding well-defined systemic conditions. These studies should identify associations with potentially predisposing and precipitating conditions. Gender differences in epidemiological studies warrant further investigation. Consensus has not been developed across the health service regarding many issues, including which facial pain problems should be treated, and when and how they should be treated.

4. The most promising approaches to management and treatment of patients with persistent pain and dysfunction may result from evidence-based practice and patient-centred care. Relaxation and cognitive behavioural therapies are effective approaches to managing chronic pain and will be discussed in Chapter 6. Further advances in diagnosis and treatment of facial pain will occur as the result of multidisciplinary collaborations among a number of fields involving basic and applied science and practice. Professional education is needed to ensure proper and safe practice in the treatment of facial pain, especially with regard to pharmacological, surgical, and behavioural approaches. Antidepressants appear to be the cheapest and most effective form of treatment.

5. There needs to be a change in clinical practice so that patients can present emotional problems without fear of rejection and clinicians can confront their own prejudices.

6. The psychological management of orofacial pain and headache requires clinicians to recognize the association between external stress, personality, and pain. It also requires changes in clinical practice so that

patients can reveal emotional problems without fear of rejection. Unfortunately, some patients will conceal both significant stress and previous psychiatric treatment. Experience and tenacity are need to obtain these essential covert details from the patient or relative. Clinicians must therefore have the training, time, and privacy to allow evaluation of emotional factors so that they will have the confidence to resist excessive investigations and surgery, and provide appropriate reassurance and treatment. Clinicians must also learn to confront their own prejudices. The concept of 'cure' must also be re-evaluated. Many patients with headache and facial pain suffer from a relapsing and recurring disorder which can be alleviated by treatment but which will often not disappear. These disorders are common, and long-term management has enormous service implications to specialist and general practitioner.

REFERENCES

Abbott, D. M. and Bush, F. M. (1991). Occlusion altered by removable appliances. *Journal of the American Dental Association*, **122**, 79.

Aghabehgi, B., Feinmann, C., and Harris, M. (1992). Prevalence of post traumatic stress disorder patients with chronic idiopathic orofacial pain. *British Journal of Oral and Maxillofacial Surgery*, **30**, 360–64.

Banks, F. R. and Kellner, M. D. (1971). Symptoms experience and health action. *Medical Care*, **9**, 498–502.

Banks, S. and Kerns, R. (1996). Explaining high rates of depression in chronic pain: a diathesis–stress framework. *Psychological Bulletin*, **119**, 95–110.

Barsky, A. J., Wood, C., and Barnett, B. M. (1994). Histories of childhood trauma in adult hypochondriacal patients. *American Journal of Psychiatry*, **1513**, 397–401.

BNF (1998) *British National Formulary*. British Medical Association and Royal Pharmaceutical Society of Great Britain, London and Oxford.

Bridges, K. and Goldberg, D. P. (1985). Somatic presentations of psychiatric illness in primary care setings. *Journal of Psychosomatic Research*, **32**, 137–44.

Brown, G. (1990). A causal relationship between life events and depression. *Journal of Abnormal Psychology*, **99**, 127–37.

Casten, R., Parmelee, P., Kleban, M., *et al.* (1995). The relationships among anxiety depression and pain in a geriatric institutional sample. *Pain*, **61**, 271–76.

Clark, T. (1984). A critical evaluation of orthopaedic occlusal appliance therapy. Design, theory and overall effectiveness. *Journal of the American Dental Association*, **108**, 359–64.

Costa, P. and MacRae, R. R. (1985). Hypochondriasis, neuroticism and ageing: when are somatic complaints unfounded? *Journal of Psychology*, **40**, 19–28.

Craig, T. K., Boardman, A. P., Mills, K., Daly-Jones, O., and Drake, H. (1993). The South London somatization study. Longitudinal course and the influence of early life experiences. *British Journal of Psychiatry*, **163**, 579–88.

DSM-IV (1994). *Diagnostic and Statistical Manual of Mental Disorders*. American Psychiatric Association.

Dworkin, R., Hartstein, G., Rosner, H. *et al.* (1992). A high-risk method for studying psycho-social antecedents of chronic pain: the prospective investigation of herpes zoster. *Journal of Abnormal Psychology*, **101**, 200–5.

Feinmann, C. (1985). The role of antidepressants in pain. *Pain*, **10**, 137–45.

Feinmann, C. (1993). The long term outcome of facial pain treatment. *Journal of Psychosomatic Research*, **37**, 381–7.

Feinmann, C. and Bass, C. (1989). The limitations of psychiatric diagnosis in the management of chronic pain. In *Human psychopharmacology. Measure and methods*, Vol. 2, (ed. P. D. Stonier and I. Hindmarch), pp. 219–34. Wiley, New York.

Feinmann, C. and Harris, M. (1984*a*). Psychogenic facial pain. Part 1. The clinical presentation. *British Dental Journal*, **156**, 165–68.

Feinmann, C. and Harris, M. (1984*b*). Psychogenic facial pain. Part 2. Management and prognosis. *British Dental Journal*, **156**, 205–8.

Feinmann, C. and Madland, G. (1998). Clinical management of orofacial pain: a multidisciplinary problem. *Current Review of Pain*, **2**, 208–16.

Franks, A. S. T. (1965). Conservative treatment of temporomandibular disorder. *Dental Practitioner*, **15**, 205–11.

Gaske, L. and O' Dowde, T. (1989). Treatment of somatisation: teaching techniques of reattribution. *Journal of Psychsomatic Research*, **33**, 697–703.

Gatchel, R., Garofalo, J., Ellis, E. *et al.* (1996). Major psychological disorders in acute and chronic TMD: an initial examination. *Journal of American Dental Association*, **127**, 1365–74.

Goldberg, R. (1994). Childhood abuse, depression and chronic pain. *Clinical Journal of Pain*, **109**; 277–81.

Green, C. and Laskin, P. (1972). Splint therapy for the MPP syndrome. *Journal of the American Dental Association*, **84**, 246–48.

Green, C. S., Mohl, N. D., McNeil, C., *et al.* (1998). Temporomandibular disorders and science. A response to the critics. *Journal of Prosthetic Dentistry*, **80**, 214–15.

Griffiths, R. H. (1983). Report on the President's Conference on the examination, diagnosis and management of temporomandibular disorders. *Journal of the American Dental Association*, **106**, 75–7.

Guthrie, E. (1996). Emotional disorders in chronic illness. Psychotherapeutic intervention. *British Journal of Psychiatry*, **168**, 265–73.

Hahn, S. B., Thompson, K., Wills, T. *et al.* (1994). The difficult doctor–patient relationship: somatisation, personality and psychopathology. *Journal of Clinical Epidemiology*, **6**, 447–657.

Harrison, S., Glover, L., Feinmann, C., *et al.* (1997). A comparison of antidepressants alone and in combination with CBT. In *Proceedings of the Eighth World Congress of Pain*, (ed. T. Jesson and J. Turner), International Association Study of Pain. IASP Press. pp. 633–43.

Heloe, B., Tieberg, A. N., and Krogstad, B. S. (1980). A multiprofessional study of patients with myofacial pain dysfunction syndrome. *Acta Odontalgia Scandinavica*, **38**, 107–17.

Horowitz, M., Wiker, N. Awarez, W., *et al.* (1979). Impact of event scale: a measure of subjective stress. *Psychosomatic Medicine*, **41**, 209–18.

Hottof, M. (1998). Occupational factors and unexplained physical symptoms. *Advances in Psychiatric Treatment*, **3**, 151–8.

Jung, A. C., Staiger, L., and Sullivan, M. (1997). The efficacy of selective serotonin re-uptake inhibitors for the management of chronic pain. *Journal of General Internal Medicine*, **12**, 384–9.

Katon, W., Von Korff, M., Lin, E. *et al.* (1990). Distressed high utiliser of medical care. *General Hospital Psychiatry*, **12**, 355–62.

Kellner, R. (1986). Maintaining factors iatrogenic reinforcement. In *Somatisation and hypochondriasis*, pp 107–111. Praeger Publishers, New York.

Korzun, A., Hinderstein, B., and Wong, M. (1996). Comorbidity of depression with chronic facial pain and temporomandibular disorders. *Oral Surgery, Oral Medicine and Oral Pathology*, **82**, 496–500.

Lascelles, R. G. (1966). Atypical facial pain and depression. *British Journal of Psychiatry*, **112**, 651–9.

Lipton, J. A. and Marbach, J. J. (1984). Predictors of treatment outcomes in patients with myofacial dysfunction syndrome. *Journal of Prosthetic Dentistry*, **51**, 387–93.

Lipton, J. A., Ship, J. A., Leresche, L., and Robinson, D. (1993). Estimated prevalence and dysfunction of reported orofacial pain in the US. *Journal of the American Dental Association*, **124**, 115–21.

McCracken, L., Gross, R., Sorg, P. *et al.* (1993). Prediction of pain in patients with chronic low back pain: effects of inaccurate prediction and pain-related anxiety. *Behaviour, Research and Therapy*, **31**, 647–52.

Magni, G. (1987). On the relationship between chronic pain and depression where there is no organic lesion. *Pain*, **31**, 1–21.

Magni, G., Moreschi, C., Rigatti-Luchini, S. *et al.* (1994). Prospective study on the relationship between depressive symptoms and chronic musculoskeletal pain. *Pain*, **56**, 289–97.

Marbach, J., Lennon, M. C., and Dohrenwend, B. (1988). Candidate risk factors for temporomandibular pain and dysfunction syndrome: psychosocial health behaviour, physical illness and injury. *Pain*, **34**, 189–51.

Mayou, R., Feinmann, C., and Hodgson, G. (1990). The present state of consultation liaison psychiatry. *Psychiatric Bulletin*, **14**, 321–5.

Mayou, R., Bass, C., and Sharpe, M. (1995). Overview of epidemiology, classification and aetiology. In *Treatment of functional somatic symptoms*, (ed. R. Mayou, C. Bass, and M. Sharpe), pp. 42–65. Oxford University Press., Oxford.

Morley, S. and Pallin, V. (1995). Scaling the affective domain of pain: a study of the dimensionality of verbal descriptors. *Pain*, **62**, 39–49.

Nemeroff, C., Vane, C. L., Phan, D., and Pollock, P. G. (1996). New anti-depressants and the cytochrome P450 system. *American Journal of Psychiatry*, **3**, 311–20.

NIH (1996). *Management of temporomandibular disorders*. National Institutes of Health, Technology Assessment Statement. NIH, Bethesda.

Oakley, M. E., McCreary, C. P., Flack, V. F., *et al.* (1989). Dentists' ability to detect psychological problems in patients with temporomandibular disorders and chronic pain. *Journal of the American Dental Association*, **118**, 727–30.

Okeson, J. P. (1996). *Orofacial Pain. Guidelines for assessment, diagnosis and management*. The American Academy of Orofacial Pain. Quintessence Books, USA.

Onghena, P. and Van Houdenhove, B. (1992). Antidepressant-induced analgesia in chronic malignant pain: A meta analysis of 39 placebo controlled studies. *Pain*, **49**, 205–19.

Orbach, R. and Dworkin, S. F. (1998). Five year outcomes in TMD relationship of changes in pain to changes in physical and psychological variables. *Journal of the American Dental Association*, **77**, 1–12.

Ramano, J. and Turner, J. (1985). Chronic pain and depression: does the evidence support a relationship? *Psychological Bulletin*, **77**, 18–34.

Ramfjord, S. P. and Ash, M. M. Jr (1995). *Occlusion*, (4th edn). W. B. Saunders, Philadelphia.

Raphael, L. and Marbach, J. (1997). Evidence based care of musculoskeletal facial pain. *Journal of American Dental Association*, **128**, 73–9.

Royal College of Physicians (1989). *Joint Working Party of the Royal College of Physicians, Psychiatrists and General Practitioners: The psychological care of medical patients*. Royal College of Physicians, London.

Shan, S. C. and Yun, W. H. (1991). Influence of an occlusal splint on integrated electromyography of the masseter muscles. *Journal of Oral Rehabilitation*, **18**, 253–8.

Shepherd, J. (1997). Tackling violence. *British Medical Journal*, **21**, 13–16.

Speculand, B., Hughes, A. O., and Gross, A. N. (1984). The role of stressful life experience in the onset of temporomandibular joint dysfunction pain. *Community Dentistry and Oral Epidemiology*, **12**, 197–202.

Turk, D. C., Zaki, H. S., and Rudy, R. E. (1993). Effects of intraoral appliance and biofeedback/stress management alone and in combination in treating pain and depression in patients with temporomandibular disorders. *Journal of Prosthetic Dentistry*, **70**, 158–64.

Turk, D., Okifuji, A., and Scharff, L. (1995). Chronic pain and depression: role of perceived impact and control in different age cohorts. *Pain*, **61**, 93–101.

Vimpari, S., Knuuttila, M., Sakki. T. *et al.* (1995). Depressive symptoms associated with symptoms of the temporomandibular joint pain dysfunction syndrome. *Psychosomatic Medicine*, **57**, 439–44.

Zautra, A., Marbach, J., Raphael, K., *et al.* (1995). The examination of myofascial face pain and its relationship to psychological distress among women. *Health Psychology*, **4**, 223–31.

5

Psychological issues in dentistry

Lesley Glover, Stephanie Jones, and Sheelah Harrison

Mike is a 34-year-old middle manager with pain in the jaw and face which radiates up to the temples. It aches and is worse in the evening and sometimes in the day. It can last for several days but is often better on a Sunday. Mike has come to your clinic for the third time complaining of this problem, you have already carried out all reasonable dental investigations and can find no evidence of organic pathology. What next?

THEORETICAL BACKGROUND

Psychology in chronic facial pain

Historically it has been accepted that the experience of pain has a psychological component. Gamsa (1994) recounts Tuke's description in 1884 of a butcher who, following an accident, was suspended by the arm on a meat hook. He yelled in pain when his sleeve was cut off to allow his arm to be examined, but when it was examined it was discovered that his arm was uninjured as the hook had only gone through his coat. Over the years other examples of the influence of psychological and situational factors have been quoted, but it was not until the mid 1960s that an explanation was proposed that included both psychological and physical factors in mechanisms underlying pain experience. Melzack and Wall's (1965) gate-control theory of pain suggested that gating mechanisms in the dorsal horns of the spinal cord modulate the flow of neural impulses from the periphery to the brain. Importantly, they suggested that these gates could be influenced by both ascending and descending pathways, thus firmly establishing psychological factors as having a role in all pain experience and recognizing that pain is complex and multiply determined.

Pain theorists now accept that whenever an individual experiences pain he will inevitably have an emotional, a cognitive, and a physical response to this pain (Melzack and Wall 1965; Skevington 1995). In turn, the nature of this response will, to a greater or lesser extent, influence his experience of pain (Melzack and Wall 1965).

Acute versus chronic pain

Despite the acknowledgement of the role of psychological factors in pain, both the general public and healthcare professionals tend to think of pain in terms of a biomedical model. In other words, pain is seen in terms of cause and effect, with physical injury or disease acting as the cause and a 'direct line transmission' of resulting pain messages producing the effect of pain. This model has much in common with an acute pain model (Hanson and Gerber 1990) which identifies pain as a temporary warning signal of physical injury or disease. The appropriate response to such a warning signal is to seek cure for the problem via medical or dental help. In cases of acute pain such help is usually available, treatment is given, and patients feel satisfied with their care. Although chronic pain is commonly though of as acute pain which persists, it differs in that often it has no underlying pathology nor can it be cured (Hanson and Gerber 1990).

In situations where pain is acute, certain behavioural responses are adaptive, for example, resting up, not using the muscles of that area, letting people know you are in pain. When pain becomes chronic (longer than 3 months), many of these responses can become at best unhelpful, and at worst harmful. A number of factors will contribute to the development of such responses, these include past experiences, the nature and extent of pain, and the approach of those around, both family and friends and healthcare professionals.

Several psychological factors will influence patients' perceptions of pain and it may be helpful to bear these in mind when faced with this problem. Anxiety and depression often worsen with pain, so the patient may be experiencing these symptoms and thus the problem is complicated still further. These patients may attend to their pain so much so that it can be difficult for them to hear what you are saying, or retain what you have said. Patients will often present with differing degrees of control over their pain. For instance, some may feel unable to carry on working whereas others feel better if they are working because it distracts them. There is no right or wrong way of dealing with pain, but some ways may be more adaptive than others. Some families may deal with pain by not talking about it, while in other families all topics of conversation might revolve around pain. Relatives and friends might encourage, discourage, or act neutrally around the person in pain. The situation will also determine the person's pain reactions. For instance, a patient who is about to complete an important and rewarding project might not notice their pain quite so much as someone who is out of work and not engaged in any hobbies. Lastly, culture might determine how tolerated a person's pain is and so influence pain behaviour, in the same way as grief is expressed differently depending on cultural mores. There is a wide variety in presentation of pain but it is generally easier, especially in the middle of a busy clinic, to view pain patients unsympathetically.

Idiopathic pain

Idiopathic or unexplained pain presents a challenge for patients and healthcare professionals in terms of understanding what exactly is happening. The majority of our upbringing and experience leads us to believe that pain does not occur without an organic cause. It has, however, been documented that the relationship between identifiable disease and chronic pain is highly variable. Tissue damage does not correlate with pain intensity as the 'direct line transmission' theory once purported, indeed such linear thinking could not explain the placebo effect or individuals' ability to tolerate ritualistic tissue damage. This is now recognized in clinical practice; for example, tension headache is diagnosed by excluding the presence of disease (Hanson and Gerber 1990), while it has been shown that there is poor correlation between radiological evidence of cervical disc degeneration and reported pain (Hanson and Gerber 1990). Without an identifiable cause it is often assumed that pain does not exist or must be imaginary. Patients are often told that 'nothing is wrong', this is, or course, entirely at odds with their experience.

In the past a psychogenic model has been used to explain the presence of idiopathic symptoms (for example, Engel 1959). This model sees pain as an emotional defence against unconscious psychic conflict. It is, however, a difficult model to test empirically and one which is reductionist in terms of ignoring possible physiological changes that are likely to accompany pain experience. Despite these criticisms it is still mistakenly used to explain idiopathic pain and the failure of medical or surgical treatments. When suggested to patients, who are experiencing their pain in physical terms, it can feel invalidating and blaming.

Lennon *et al.* (1989) described individuals experiencing chronic idiopathic facial pain as feeling stigmatized. In a study of 151 patients with temporomandibular pain and dysfunction syndrome, they reported that the majority felt estranged from others and misunderstood because of their facial pain. They found that stigma perceptions were positively associated with the number of different medical specialists consulted for pain and with having been told by a doctor that the pain is all imaginary. In a more recent study, Garro (1994) analysed the narrative representations of chronic illness experience of 32 patients with temporomandibular joint dysfunction. Emerging themes focused on the attempt of patients to make sense of their symptoms within the framework of mind–body dualism and on patients' search for an answer that would help them to make sense of what was happening to them.

These studies highlight the need for patients to have an explanation of their symptoms or illness which fits with their own experience and which makes sense in terms of their general understanding of pain. If they and their healthcare practitioner hold an acute model of pain, then the presenting features of chronic idiopathic facial pain will not make sense to either of them. This lack of a clear explanation will increase patient distress (and the clinician's, see below) and is likely to lead to an increased focus on symptoms. A vicious circle can be established whereby distress and pain watching in turn increase the subjective experience of pain and lead to more distress, and so on.

The notion that there is no identifiable or treatable pathology rather than no physical change is often not made clear to patients. They may be left feeling misunderstood or disbelieved. They may feel that information or treatment is being withheld for financial or punitive reasons. Alternatively, they may think that if the doctor or dentist understood the extent of their pain they would never leave them in that state but would provide necessary treatment to alleviate their suffering. Both these sets of ideas set up a situation where the patient feels that he needs to prove his case to the doctor in order to gain help. Such a situation is extremely unhelpful and can usually be avoided with careful handling. In order to achieve this, it is necessary to have an understanding of the underlying constructions of the problem held by both patient and professional. These two then need to go on to develop a shared model and a common goal (see below) .

The biopsychosocial model of pain (Engel 1977) acknowledges the role of psychological, behavioural, and social factors in the patient's experience as well as physical factors. This model helps to avoid a reductionist focus on physical processes and treatments, and encourages an holistic approach to the care of patients with chronic pain. It can help patients make sense of what is happening to them and can provide an indication of the type and range of intervention which may be helpful.

PATIENT MANAGEMENT

Psychology in dentistry/primary care

Dentists are used to employing psychological techniques to help patients cope with the stress of investigation and treatment. They are skilled in treating anxious patients and in minimizing potential distress. For example, dentists are often taught to use non-emotive, non-pain words to help relax patients and increase their ability to manage painful procedures, they might say 'you might feel a stinging' or 'this will feel cold' rather than 'this will hurt'. These kinds of psychological techniques are different from those needed to manage patients presenting at the surgery in distress about a problem which may not be curable; however, some skills, particularly those in managing anxiety, will be transferable.

It has already been described that this group of patients may be very distressed. Levels of distress will vary and some patients may need specialist psychological help in managing their pain while others can be managed in a primary-care setting. This section examines the management of patients in primary care and suggest how to judge when referral to psychology or psychiatry is necessary. Different dentists will want to be more or less involved. Some will want to do the minimum, while others will have a greater interest (or greater resources) in addressing psychosocial care for these patients. Later in this section, a two-stage approach is outlined. Stage one is basic 'in-house' management, while stage two provides scope for identifying and addressing psychosocial issues in more detail. Communication issues will be considered next.

Communication in the consultation

Often problems arise, as suggested earlier, from poor communication between doctor and patient which leads to a lack of shared understanding of what is happening. Also in the dynamic may be feelings of inadequacy on the part of professionals who are trained to identify pathology and fix it. Where idiopathic pains are concerned, this is not possible and this can make pain patients unattractive to manage. It has been well documented that at the best of times communication between doctor and patient is poor. Ley (1988) suggests that only a small proportion of information given is retained following consultation in general practice. Information about diagnosis and treatment is often poorly remembered even when the information may be unambiguous and anticipated. A mismatch between patient and professional understanding of the situation means that even less information will be retained.

To gain a thorough understanding of the patient's problem it is necessary to use skills to elicit information. This is often time consuming, but any attempt to hurry may, in the end, extend the process and increase the number of consultations. The approach used will also impact on the patient and contribute to his emotional and behavioural response. Counselling skills are useful, so listen and reflect, use open questions, express warmth, respect, genuineness, and empathy (Rogers 1961).

Diagnostic feedback

Patients attending for results may be thinking the worst and will be eager to hear the diagnosis. However, hearing that they do not have a recognized problem may increase their anxiety. For many patients a diagnosis is helpful because it validates the subjective experience and tells them that their condition is recognizable and they are not the only person to have experienced it. It may also increase hope, reduce distress, and provide social legitimacy. For many patients with facial pain who fell isolated and misunderstood a diagnosis can be invaluable. However, where a diagnosis is not easily made, it may be more helpful not to speculate, as patients can become preoccupied with the meaning, have certain expectation of symptoms, and anticipate future disability (Williams 1996). What is said and how definitely the diagnosis is stated (e.g. unexplained pain, atypical facial pain, or chronic idiopathic facial pain) will depend on a number of factors and will affect patient responses. Thomas (1987) found that a positive consultation (a firm diagnosis) rather than a negative one (no diagnosis) resulted in a higher proportion of improvement in patients attending general practice with cold, pain, and fatigue symptoms. Having an explanation which provided reassurance and information about a possible prognosis seems to have been helpful to this cohort. Whatever is said, it is important to normalize the patient's problems; for example, 'this is a common condition from which many patients suffer; it is the next most common form of facial pain after dental pain'.

Although it can feel very difficult to say 'I don't know what's wrong', patients often value honesty. Where a diagnosis is unknown it may be possible to give definite information as to what is *not* wrong. However, given that it may be that this is not what is happening, it is conceivable that the patient may not be wholly reassured. 'Holding' their anxieties by recognizing that they are understandably anxious and, where possible, reassuring them that 'every feasible test has been done so that it is clear it is not an abscess or cancer' will be a valuable part of management.

Also important in containing patient anxieties is the provision of understandable information. Give an explanation about the possible physiological processes involved, remembering to tailor it to an appropriate level of understanding (see Ley (1988) for more on helpful ways of relaying information). Giving information needs to be balanced with the patient's view of what is happening to him/her; it is advisable to spend some time comparing your explanation with the patient's own beliefs. Ask the patient what s/he has understood from the explanation, ensure that s/he has grasped the key points and find out how the explanation sounds to him/her. Some patients are able to accept the termination of investigations and treatments, but others may feel angry and let down, whether or not they express this.

The 'psychogenic' issue

Having heard that you cannot name their pain or cure it, many patients will conclude that you think they are making it up. They may or may not verbalize this. Possibly the most important point is not to say, or even suggest, that there is nothing wrong—there obviously is or the patient would not have pain—whatever your aetiological hypothesis. In fact, if there is no *identifiable* pathology an explanation may be 'Using the scientific tests that are currently available, no problems show'. In order to pre-empt the problems this assumption will cause, introduce the issues, for example 'some patients think, when told there is no problem, that they are imagining it but many patients have pain for which no identifiable cause is found'.

Integrating medical and psychosocial perspectives

Once all possible dental pathology has been excluded, it is necessary to take a broader view of the situation and begin to examine possible psychological and social factors which may be contributing to the experience of physical pain. The purpose of this is to assess whether there is room to improve the patient's condition by the introduction of self-management strategies (such a broad view may be appropriate anyway regardless of treatability of the problem). With this biopsycho-social model in mind, a two-stage approach to managing patients in primary care is suggested.

Stage one

In addition to counselling skills, there are a number of key elements that will inform your discussion when managing these patients 'in house'. If patients feel understood, they can channel their energy into coping rather than convincing health professionals that there is something wrong with them. Information-giving involves a two-way conversation and Ley (1988) discussed the evidence for effective communication with patients. Show understanding by gauging the patient's expectations, 'What are you hoping for today?', and try to empathize with their experience of pain. Many patients will have their own theory of what is happening to them and to help understand their perspective a question may be, 'What are your ideas about your pain?'.

Listening to what patients are saying and providing informed reassurance is an effective intervention strategy. In a recent trial, 40 per cent of patients with pain attending for assessment in a specialist facial pain clinic opted for no treatment following reassurance (Harrison 1996).

Having pain for which there seems no reasonable explanation makes managing the pain much harder than if its presence makes sense, for example 'I overdid it at keep fit last night'. Once the cause of pain has been discussed, the patient may be keen to know what treatment is offered. A lack of curative treatment may be disappointing. Western medicine has long touted the notion that doctors cure suffering; doctors and dentists feel strongly that their role should be curative, even when they do not have the answers.

Prognostic information, for example 'Most people find the pain gets better on its own; however, for some people it can come and go. You may find it takes a little time to go away', may be helpful. It is important to be honest and this should be balanced with giving hope where possible.

Discuss the possibility for symptomatic treatment (for example analgesic medication, antidepressants) but be aware of possible side-effects and contraindications. The patient's desire for improvement in their condition may compel them to try any treatment, 'I'll try anything'. Ultimately symptomatic treatment might make things worse, and so again 'holding' their anxiety and being empathic will minimize possibly detrimental treatment-seeking behaviour. For example, if patients are experiencing tooth pain they may put pressure on you to remove a healthy tooth. Unless you have evidence that the tooth is damaged is some way, this is to be resisted as it will not help pain and may exacerbate it . Explaining clearly the reason for not extracting a tooth is important, to minimize the chance of patients seeking such treatment elsewhere.

Address follow-up; if you do not arrange another appointment, make it clear that patients can come back and see you if necessary. By leaving the door open, patients are less likely to feel the need to use it. Also, providing written information if you have it facilitates the processing of information and shows the patients that they are not suffering from an unknown condition (see Mayberry and Mayberry (1996) for guidelines on writing a leaflet).

Stage two

If patients return after stage one (either planned or unplanned), then it may be prudent to conduct a fuller assessment to judge the necessity of referral on to other services. There are guidelines on the use of this assessment method within the primary-care setting (Sullivan *et al.* 1991). Individuals can not be thought of without considering the context in which they live. It may be that they have had pain for some time but because of their current circumstances that pain has become unmanageable. Alternatively, they may perceive a physical symptom as the only thing over which they can gain some control in a chaotic or stressed life. The reason for presenting is important, as is the question 'why now?'.

Begin this second-stage assessment with pain-related questions and move from there to other issues via the route 'How has pain affected your life?'. A sensitive approach is necessary if it is to be possible to create a relationship with the patient where social and psychological factors can be explored without the patient feeling intruded on or that the questions are inappropriate. When attending the dentist for toothache or jaw ache it is not perceived as usual, necessary, or appropriate to be asked about relationships, etc., and yet if these issues are explored in an appropriate way within the context of coping with pain, it can be invaluable and limits the possibility of patients sensing that you think they are imagining the pain. It is important to get across the message that the patient is not being fobbed off but that medical management is not effective in this problem so the emphasis needs to change to one of self-management.

Try to examine all aspects of the pain. The diagnostic interview will have generated information, but over and above site of pain, duration, precipitating and relieving factors, it is necessary to find out in more detail when it began, what else was happening at the time, and how it began. Ask about patterns of pain, its antecedents and consequences. Find out 'What makes the pain better?' and 'What makes the pain worse?' and whether patients are ever distracted from their pain by an absorbing activity. Helping patients clarify these issues may aid them in recognizing ways that they can maximize their coping.

Equally, asking about home situation, about activities, and what they may have stopped because of the pain may lead into a discussion of losses such as mobility, independence, work, finances, or role. These are all integral aspects of a person's identity and loss of them may be adversely affecting the patient's mood. Allowing discussion of changes resulting from pain facilitates the expression of tensions. This is particularly important because it might be exacerbating pain. Assess mood and, if worryingly low, refer and manage appropriately.

While this sounds like a lot of information, and it may not be possible to gather it all, even gaining some will help in understanding the impact of pain on their lives and may guide you in what to do next. Importantly, it will also serve to help the patient feel understood.

Referring on

Clearly the referral should be discussed and agreed upon with the patient. Outline in brief what psychological pain management is all about and give the patient some idea of what to expect from the assessment. Think about the meaning that the referral may have for an individual. For example, it may indicate to him that he is not disbelieved. In pain management services, patients often arrive for assessment in a very hostile, angry frame of mind because they assume the referral is made because the referrer thinks their pain is all in the mind or, worse still (but not uncommon), because it suggests to them that they might be going mad. It can be helpful to say something like 'If pain was easy to cope with, people would manage with no problem, but it is not easy and therefore people often need help to deal with it'.

If it appears that a patient's strategies to cope with his pain are limited or are not working, then referral to a clinical psychology or pain management service may be appropriate. This kind of referral may be accessible through a specialist pain management centre or a general psychology department. Alternatively, the GP may have information about local services. This treatment will entail a number of interventions, including stress management, relaxation and hypnotic visualization training, behavioural and cognitive therapy. Details about these interventions are covered in Chapter 6.

In more severe cases, a psychiatric referral may be advisable, most often if the patient is suicidal or showing signs of psychosis.

For some patients who are managing reasonably well, attending local classes in relaxation, stress management, or assertiveness training may prove helpful in enabling them to improve their quality of life, and may be more acceptable than referring on.

Potential difficulties in managing pain patients

Some patients who present with excessive health anxieties may be angry or cynical, while at the other end of the spectrum are patients who may be relieved to hear that there is no treatable organic cause. However patients present, there are common concerns and problems frequently encountered by health workers in this area.

It is important to ask questions about psychosocial problems. Patients with long-standing pain might well be sensitive even to the remotest hint that they are making up the pain, that it is not real, or that they are depressed and this is causing the pain. Perhaps they have heard this from doctors, friends, etc. Such a history increases the need for a sensitive approach and it may be necessary to state quite plainly that they have real pain.

It is likely that the majority may not have had the opportunity to express their thoughts and feelings about their pain, or may not have discussed it with friends and family for fear of being seen as moaning or mad. They may therefore feel a need to talk about their pain, and the distress of this can open up many difficult, personal, and unresolved issues. If the patient does need to talk and time is insufficient, they may be told that this is not the right place to go into detail, and in this or future appointments discuss the possibility of counselling. If the pain talk continues unabated, this may be because it has not been acknowledged sufficiently or the patient has not communicated sufficiently how bad his pain is.

Patients may deny, ignore, or even disbelieve a doctor who says he cannot cure their pain. Related to this denial may be an apparently logical request to continue the medical intervention. Indeed it may seems to them that the only sensible step is to continue looking for the cause of their pain. This might mean having more tests and/or consulting other practitioners. Although a reasonable amount of investigation and opinion should be sought, there may come a point at which this is counterproductive or even harmful. Good rapport with patients may encourage them to tell you of such plans and give you the opportunity to suggest more appropriate routes of referral; for example, a centre specializing in the treatment of chronic idiopathic facial pain.

Chronic pain is a debilitating and distressing problem for the patient and can be difficult for the professional. When managing such patients a range of emotion, including annoyance and feelings of failure, may be felt. In addition, you may be affected by patients' distress, thus making the interaction quite different from a usual consultation. Be aware of this, and if choosing to become more involved, make appropriate links with specialist services and use informal networks for support. Do not underestimate the demands that will be made on personal resources.

SUMMARY

Do:

- reassure;
- listen to beliefs about what is going on.

Don't:

- reassure again and again and again;
- let patients think you think their pain is imaginary;
- feel pressurized to come up with a diagnosis or cure if there isn't one.

REFERENCES

Engel, G. L. (1959). 'Psychogenic' pain and pain-prone patient. *American Journal of Medicine*, **26**, 899–918.

Engel, G. L. (1977). The need for a new medical model. *Science*, **196**, 129–36.

Engel, G. L. (1980). The clinical application of the biopsychosocial model. *American Jounal of Psychiatry*, **137**, (5), 535–44

Gamsa, A. (1994). The role of psychological factors in chronic pain. *Pain*, **57**, 5–29.

Garro, L. C. (1994). Narrative representations of chronic illness experience: cultural models of illness in mind and body in stories concerning the temporomandibular joint (TMJ). *Social Sciences and Medicine*, **38**, 775–7.

Hanson, R. W. and Gerber, K. E. (1990). *Coping with chronic pain: a guide to patient self-management*. Guildford Press, New York.

Harrison, S., Glover, L., and Miles, A. (1996) Do treatment trials recruit representative samples? *Proceedings of the British Psychological Society*, **4**, 58.

Lennon, M. C., Link, B. G., Marbach, J. J., and Dohrenwend, B. P. (1989). The stigma of chronic facial pain and its impact on social relationships. *Social Problems*, **36**, (2), 117–33.

Ley, P. (1988). *Communicating with patients*. Chapman & Hall, London.

Mayberry, J.C. and Mayberry, M. (1996). Effective instructions for patients. *Journal of the Royal College of Physicians of London*, **30**, 206–8.

Melzack, R. and Wall, P. D. (1965). Pain mechanisms: a new theory. *Science*, **50**, 971–9.

Rogers, C. R. (1961). *On becoming a person*. Houghton Miffin, Boston.

Skevington, S. M. (1995). *Psychology of pain*. Wiley, Chicester.

Sullivan, M. D., Turner, J. A., and Romano, J. (1991). Chronic pain in primary care. Identification and management of psychosocial factors. *Journal of Family Practice*, **32**, 193–9.

Thomas, K. B. (1987). General practice consultations: is there any point in being positive? *British Medical Journal*, **294**, 1200–2.

Williams, A. C. de C. (1996). Can a diagnosis be disadvantageous? *Health Psychology Update*.

6

Cognitive behaviour therapy in the management of chronic idiopathic facial pain

Stephanie Jones, Lesley Glover, and Sheelah Harrison

The aim of this chapter is to provide information about the theory and practice of cognitive behaviour therapy (CBT) and its application to the management of facial pain. It is a summary of a clinical psychology intervention and not a 'manual' for clinicians not trained in CBT. In the first part, cognitive behavioural interventions are introduced, then the application to treatment of pain is described, before finishing with a description of the techniques most often used.

PSYCHOLOGICAL TREATMENT

Cognitive behaviour therapy is usually a brief psychological therapy that is concerned principally with overcoming identified problems and achieving specific targets. The aim of CBT is to enable people to manage their difficulties by applying researched principles of thoughts, feelings, and behaviour. These principles translate into practical strategies which can lead to changes in subjective and objective thoughts, feelings, and behaviour states. The approach is characterized by its structured treatment sessions and the collaborative relationship between patient and therapist. Treatment is based on theoretically and pragmatically well-founded techniques which are applied selectively to each individual case as needed.

Although there is some evidence for the efficacy of brief dynamic psychotherapy in refractory irritable bowel syndrome (Guthrie and Creed 1991), CBT is the most commonly practised therapy. It is also the best supported by evidence from randomized trials, for example in non-cardiac chest pain (Klimes *et al.* 1990), patients with medically unexplained symptoms (Speckens *et al.* 1995), and in chronic fatigue syndrome (Sharpe *et al.* 1996).

THE DEVELOPMENT OF CBT

The most commonly used approach in the management of pain, CBT, is derived from the combination of behaviour therapy and cognitive theory.

Behaviourism

Behavioural science began early in the twentieth century with studies of animal learning by early psychologists (e.g. Pavlov and Skinner), who showed that behaviour could be predicted and manipulated by external situations and events. Using knowledge of this they came to recognize a series of contingencies which guided behaviour and therefore could be deliberately modified to alter behaviour.

Furthermore, responses were partially contingent upon the reinforcement or punishment received from the environment. Later extension of the stimulus–response model began to account for the more complex interaction of the response (behaviour), which could itself determine the stimulus. The work of social learning theorists challenged the simple behavioural theories by demonstrating that behaviour could be modified through learning.

Gamsa's (1994) review of the theoretical development in psychological pain management suggests that behaviour theory is commensurate with the sensory model of pain physiology. That is, the experience of pain is a response to sensory stimuli which are influenced by external factors and could seemingly reinforce or extinguish pain. However, as theories of pain developed it was possible to begin to explain the much more complicated behaviour apparent in chronic pain. This appears to be a multiply determined behaviour resulting from the interaction between the individual and the environment (family, society, etc.). For example, pain may cause a patient to avoid an activity, thereby lowering perceived pain which, in turn, stimulates another person to increase their activity, which then serves to reinforce the patient's lower level of activity and strengthen the association between low activity and pain reduction.

Cognitive science

With the advent of cognitive science, coming as it did on the heels of psychoanalysis, behavioural explanations were extended to acknowledge the role of mental and emotional factors in behaviour. A number of psychologists, of whom Aaron Beck is unquestionably the most influential, began to consider the role of thoughts and beliefs in the development and maintenance of psychological problems.

Beck began by using his theory to explain how depression (Beck 1967), low mood, and problematic behaviour are the consequence of negative thinking patterns. Negative thinking is the result of cognitive processing which translates external events into internal representations. Beck suggested that it was the internal representations rather than the events themselves which determined conscious cognition and subsequent mood state.

The depressed individual displays systematic errors in thought processes which lead to negative conclusions. These errors include: overgeneralization (translation of a negative experience into a general rule), personalization, dichotomous thinking (seeing things in an 'either/or' way), and selective abstraction (noticing negative experiences and ignoring or discounting positive ones). Specific distorted styles vary between individuals but they usually occur without conscious awareness and have been termed negative automatic thoughts.

Depressed individuals' thoughts revolve around themes of loss, including loss in relation to the self (seeing the self as inadequate and unworthy), the world (perceiving oneself as being deprived of external sources of pleasure), and the future (anticipating general bleakness and lack of success). Together these themes are referred to as the negative cognitive triad.

Underlying the cognitive triad is a set of basic beliefs, attitudes, or premises which are maladaptive. Ongoing experience is evaluated using these sets of beliefs, which are referred to as schemata. Depressogenic schemata would typically include a number of attitudes such as, 'I must do everything perfectly' or 'Everyone must like me'. Any evidence that challenges these premises is a threat to the individual's belief system and therefore results in a loss of self-esteem. Beck suggested that sensitizing experiences in early life led to negative views of the self, world, and future, and that these lead to dormant depressogenic cognitive schemata.

The experience of pain is a negative one and commonly patients with chronic pain have negative automatic thoughts relating specifically to their pain and, as a consequence, to life more generally. For instance, thoughts such as 'I can't cope' will lead to distress and feelings of hopelessness. In addition they do not encourage coping behaviours. When the thought is modified to the usually more accurate 'I don't want to have to cope with this pain but I have coped before and I will be able to now', the individual can begin to think about what might be helpful and take appropriate action.

The combination of cognitive and behaviour therapy has led to the treatment approach labelled CBT. The following sections will examine the practice and evaluation of CBT in chronic facial pain.

THE PRACTICE OF COGNITIVE BEHAVIOUR THERAPY
FOR CHRONIC FACIAL PAIN

The initial assessment lasts between one and three appointments and may be about 1 hour long. Towards the end, the clinical psychologist and patient will discuss possible treatment options. If CBT is selected, aims and objectives and a set period of treatment, between 6 and 20 sessions, are agreed.

The assessment is a semi-structured interview covering the immediate problems and the history and development of the problem. It is sensible to begin with the impact of pain on current life style as this will be uppermost on the patient's mind. Patients may have ceased activities because of pain, low mood, or both. For example, a patient may not eat out in public because eating hurts his jaw, or no longer wants to go out because he is depressed. It is important to try to establish what has stopped because of pain and what has stopped because of mood.

An appraisal of the quality of the pain and what makes it better or worse can be done by asking about a 'usual pain episode' and exploring the triggers to, and consequences of, pain. The language the patient uses to describe pain, the way he describes it, or an inability to describe it, will guide the clinician in the best approach to treatment.

Patients are asked to set goals in order to return to previous activities. This is an important question because it helps assess motivation for treatment. If a patient was unable to identify any goals (despite having altered or ceased many activities), it may indicate a high level of mood disturbance, particularly low self-efficacy or an inability to resolve his difficulties. Patients may have unrealistic goals. It is useful to ask patients what life would be like without pain.

A personal and pain history improves the clinician's understanding of the patient and helps put the pain in the context of the rest of the patient's life, and the extent to which the pain has changed him. At this point the patients often express angry and disappointed feelings about loss, with the medical process, or even with specific people.

The history usually entails a brief outline of major events and milestones, any early difficulties in relation to parents and significant others, and assessment of any outstanding, substantial psychological problems that affect the patient and may require a different psychological approach.

After the developmental history, current family and social relationships are explored, for instance have other people in the family been affected by pain? If the whole family is under stress, tempers may be frayed and roles may have changed. The family may be a source of stress, or of abnormal illness beliefs, or they may reinforce the sick role. Family therapy has been advocated but not systematically evaluated for the treatment of functional somatic symptoms. However the pain is managed at home, it is likely to have an impact on the outcome of treatment. Family members will need information and it may be appropriate to involve them in treatment.

Standard psychological assessments are often used because they provide objective measures which can be used to guide treatment and evaluate outcome. The areas assessed include mood, function, self-efficacy, and coping style. For a full review of reliability and validity see Williams and Erskine (1995).

Therapist–patient relationship

During the assessment the clinical psychologist will develop a shared model of pain management with which the patient can collaborate. The ability of the patient to share a biopsychosocial view of pain is crucial, and can be determined largely in the assessment stages. The patient may be rooted in an organic explanation of pain and may fail to understand the importance of psychological factors. Treatment then has an unclear purpose and intense and difficult psychological treatment is unlikely to succeed.

The successful practice of CBT requires that the therapist cultivates a special type of relationship with the patient. This is different from the usual doctor–patient relationship and is more like that between a student and a tutor. Rather than giving didactic instructions, therapist and patient work together to discover how the patient's current thinking and behaviour may be maintaining the problem and how positive change may be brought about.

From the outset, realistic and unrealistic goals of treatment are made explicit. It is made clear that a 'cure' is unrealistic and that the treatment process requires the patient to take an active role in a collaborative working alliance. Guthrie (1995) has stressed that psychological work with patients with physical symptoms requires negotiated, realistic goals which are acceptable to patient and therapist.

The collaboration and clear communication of all healthcare professionals involved in a patient's care is of obvious importance. However, not all may hold the same view of the problem and so it may be necessary to make a contract with the patient in which he agrees not to pursue further medical consultations while he or she is receiving CBT (Salkovskis 1989).

Multidisciplinary teams

As a consequence of possible treatment components, and the type of patients being treated in a pain management programme, a multidisciplinary team consisting of a variety of specialists, including nurses, anaesthetists, physiotherapists, psychiatrists, clinical psychologists, surgeons, and physicians will manage the patient. Programmes can be individual or in groups. Patients appear to prefer individual treatments (Spence 1989) and these have the advantage that they are tailored to individual need. At present, cognitive therapy is mostly provided by clinical psychologists; however, other disciplines are now acquiring these skills and using them in a number of clinical settings, sometimes combined with other techniques, such as hypnosis.

It is important to consider how a clinical psychologist and a liaison psychiatrist interact. Their roles are complementary rather than competitive, and exact roles need to be negotiated flexibly depending on the nature of the service available. It may be appropriate for a psychiatrist to concentrate on those patients who do not do so well with group-based programmes. The most valuable interaction is probably at the point of entry into a programme.

TYPICAL CBT INTERVENTIONS

Goal setting

At the start of therapy patients are encouraged to set achievable, realistic, specific short- and long-term goals. Once identified, the patient is encouraged to achieve them in a series of steps in order to increase self-efficacy. More difficult goals can be set as self-efficacy improves.

Challenging negative automatic thoughts

A first step is to encourage patients to monitor thinking, to elicit negative pain-related automatic thoughts, and then to test and challenge such thoughts. This is achieved by questioning the accuracy of thoughts, looking for evidence to confirm or refute them, and by encouraging objective views of the problem. Once alternatives are identified, patients are encouraged to confirm these through behavioural experiments(see Hawton *et al.* (1989) for a detailed description of thought eliciting and challenging). Having challenged the thought 'I can't cope', a patient may employ a relaxation technique when pain is bad, and monitor the outcome. Addressing other thoughts about causes and consequences of pain, and whether their pain is believed, will be valuable in relieving distress, increasing self-help strategies, and preventing conflict with healthcare professionals.

Some examples of pain-related thoughts are:

- 'Life won't be worth living until the pain is gone.'

- 'I can't be happy and in pain. I'm in pain all the time, therefore I can't be happy.'
- 'If only the doctors understood how bad the pain is, they would treat me.'
- 'It can't be possible to have pain this bad unless something is very wrong.'
- 'Nobody takes me seriously.'

Relaxation and breathing strategies

Relaxation combined with diaphragmatic breathing exercises can help reduce pain. Relaxing neck, jaws, and shoulders can give transient control over pain.

Cognitive visualization strategies

Cognitive strategies are used in combination with relaxation to help distract from pain and to alter pain sensation. Visualization attempts to replace attention on pain with more pleasant information. Patients are encouraged to use one or more of a variety of active and passive visualization techniques to modify pain. Passive strategies may entail watching or listening to something interesting, focusing on a pattern, or counting, or reciting poetry. Active strategies may be imaginative distraction or imaginative relabelling. Imaginative distraction aims to replace the experiences of pain with incompatible stimuli—you can't be comfortable and in pain at the same time. An example of imaginative distraction is to imagine a warm beach and rolling waves. Imaginative relabelling means relabelling the context of the pain to a sensation which is more bearable—red hot pain becomes less red, cooled by an ice block to a cool blue.

Behavioural coping strategies

A planned, systematic programme will encourage paced activity and exercise, built up in gradual small increments in patients whose pain has forced them to abandon work, leisure activities, or socializing. It is important to prevent both over- and underactivity.

Stress management and assertion skills

Managing stress, particularly in those facial arthromyalgia (FAM) patients who make a close link between stress and pain, will reduce pain. It may be possible to relabel pain as an early warning of stress. Even if patients do not make a link between stress and pain, pain is stressful, stress is cumulative, and stress management is therefore helpful.

Box 6.1 CBT interventions

1. Goal setting.
2. Challenging negative automatic thoughts.
3. Relaxation and breathing exercises.
4. Cognitive visualization strategies.
5. Behavioural coping strategies.
6. Stress management and assertion skills.

THE EFFICACY OF CBT IN THE TREATMENT OF PAIN

CBT methods have been widely incorporated into the management of chronic pain, most often musculoskeletal conditions, and their use is now commonplace in specialist pain clinics (Dworkin *et al.* 1994). The efficacy of CBT in the treatment of chronic pain has been investigated by numerous researchers (Turner and Chapman 1982; Turk *et al.* 1983; Skinner *et al.* 1990) and clinical effectiveness has been demonstrated with a wide range of pain syndromes. Laboratory-based studies have shown the possible enhancement of pain tolerance using a CBT approach (Klepac *et al.* 1981) and clinical studies have shown favourable results in the treatment of low back pain (Hazard *et al.* 1991), arthritis (O'Leary *et al.* 1998), headaches (Holroyd *et al.* 1991), atypical chest pains (Klimes *et al.* 1990), repetitive strain injury (Spence 1989), temporomandibular joint (TMJ) pain (Olson and Malow 1987), and in numerous mixed chronic pain groups (Kerns *et al.* 1986; Skinner *et al.* 1990; Nicholas *et al.* 1992).

Two factors make it difficult to assess how effective these measures are: first, measuring outcome in this type of treatment for pain is difficult as the aim is ambiguous; and, secondly, even when the intended aim is clearer, not all pain programmes incorporate exactly the same treatments, so comparing results can be complicated. Although all CBT interventions aim to help patients identify maladaptive patterns and to acquire, develop, and practice more adaptive coping techniques, exact treatments may vary from study to study and from clinic to clinic. Pain management programme content varies and may include any number of individual components. CBT is not designed to eliminate patients' pain but to help them live with their pain more effectively. The pain may be reduced as a result of the increased activity and by means of various coping skills, but this is not an explicit aim. Consequently, given that a reduction in pain severity is unlikely to occur, it is more difficult to assess outcome. Outcome measures therefore focus on issues of quality of life, functional status, self-reported mood, and others.

There are many other problems in evaluating outcome of pain management programmes; including selection of very specific groups of patients, possibly those most likely to benefit from the interventions (Turk and Rudy 1990). One study aimed to address these issues by assessing the effectiveness of a CBT intervention in comparison with non-interventional support and medication in a routine healthcare setting. No difference could be detected between the two treatment groups, except that those having CBT showed a trend towards improvement after the treatment had ceased (Pilowsky *et al*. 1995). The study highlighted the problem of discontinuation of treatment before completion by a large number of patients (one-third), which was greater in the CBT group and suggested that a number of patients found psychological treatment uncomfortable. These treatment dropout findings have been replicated by others (Dworkin *et al*. 1994) and suggest that patient selection may be helpful in preventing this; and that this treatment is not for everybody. CBT is not a treatment which can be prescribed in the same way as medical or surgical treatments. It requires a degree of openness and commitment to a self-help approach. If patients are committed to a medical explanation and are seeking a medical or surgical cure for their pain, then psychology may not be appropriate for them at this time. One aim of the assessment is to ascertain this readiness for a psychological approach. Comparisons between different approaches and treatment are thus difficult, especially when treatment groups contain heterogeneous collections of patients. The treatment response varies for individuals, with individual psychological factors appearing to have some influence upon outcome (Tota-Faucette *et al*. 1993).

The outcome measures shown in Box 6.2 are frequently used to define success of pain management. Specific measures chosen will depend on the reason for measuring outcome: researchers may be interested in changing cognitions or coping styles; the patient may be interested in mood state; purchasers and employees in the likelihood of returning to work.

Follow-up of between 6 months and 2 years in some of the above studies has indicated that improvements may be maintained for

Box 6.2 Outcome measures frequently used to define success of pain management

- Return to work.
- Reduce medication use.
- Minimize healthcare system use.
- Stabilize mood—anxiety and depression.
- Change pain-coping styles.
- Increase self-efficacy.
- Increase feelings of control.
- Increase in activity.

considerable periods after treatment completion, and in many studies improvements have been shown to continue after the CBT has ceased (Manchini *et al*. 1988; Turner and Clancy 1988; Nicholas *et al*. 1992; Dworkin *et al*. 1994).

APPLYING CBT TO THE TREATMENT OF CHRONIC FACIAL PAIN

CBT has been widely applied in the management of chronic pain. In particular, it has been used for pain that leads to major functional impairment, e.g. back pain. Although chronic facial pain stands out from the traditional areas of pain management, in that the patients are not disabled, these patients with facial pain share some aspects of the experience of pain with other pain patients. They are distressed by their pain and often report limitation of their activities. Many of them are working but they often avoid situations. They find social occasions can be difficult, as laughing, smiling, and talking may be painful. Patients with FAM pain may avoid eating in public. Despite the unquestionable level of distress which accompanies chronic facial pain, little work has been done in using CBT intervention to help this group manage their pain.

Brief group CBT (minimal intervention therapy, as described by Glasgow *et al*. 1991) has been undertaken in TMJ pain patients and compared to 'routine treatment'. At 3 months both groups of patients had similar results, but over 12 months the CBT group continued to improve on measures of pain and the degree to which the pain interfered with their lives. Measures of somatization, depression, and mandibular opening indicated that the more dysfunctional patients did not benefit from the minimal intervention (Dworkin *et al.* 1994).

THE EFP PROJECT

In a study of the treatment of facial pain at the Eastman Dental Hospital (the EFP project), CBT was adapted and used with a large cohort of patients with chronic idiopathic facial pain (excluding trigeminal neuralgia). The adaptation focused on expanding the cognitive side of the intervention and reducing the behavioural side. Experience suggested that the main task in managing these patients was explaining the presence of pain in the absence of an identifiable cause and then reaching an acceptance that there may be no cure. This enabled attention to be turned towards a self-help approach to managing pain rather than continued seeking of medical or surgical intervention.

The EFP project provided evidence that combining drug treatment with CBT reduces the degree to which pain interferes in patients' lives and increases the control they feel over their lives after 3 months of treatment. CBT and fluoxetine were assessed alone and in combination (Harrison *et al.* 1997). The continuing study will investigate whether these changes are maintained with time.

Intervention

In order to recruit sufficient patients 900 were assessed and 120 recruited into the study. In the EFP project patients were seen for a total of six appointments, each lasting for 1 hour, at fortnightly intervals. They then had follow-up appointments at 3, 6, and 9 months following the completion of the intervention. The intervention was adapted from established pain-management programmes and contained the elements described below. All areas were addressed to a greater or lesser extent with all patients, although individual needs determined the extent to which each area was covered.

The patients had a 6-week baseline period between initial assessment and first treatment session. The facial pain clinician saw all patients monthly for the first 3 months. At each session progress was reviewed, concerns discussed, and reassurance and counselling provided. The patients also received 1 month's supply of medication, the consumption of which was monitored by the clinician. Those patients assigned to CBT had a monthly interview with the clinical psychologist during the 3-month treatment period. Patients were asked to refrain from other pain treatment and have only minimal dentistry.

Results

A comparison of fluoxetine (Prozac®) alone and in combination with CBT showed that fluoxetine reduced pain severity, and CBT and fluoxetine reduced distress and increased control. Figure 6.1 shows the median multidimensional pain inventory (MPI) scores. The MPI pain severity scores were reduced in both the drug and drug with CBT groups. The MPI interference with life scores improved in all groups except placebo only. Patients' life control scores were increased in both CBT treatment groups. Psychological distress, measured by the MPI, was reduced in the drug alone and the drug plus CBT groups. Pain severity and distress measured by the MPI were positively correlated with distress.

These results are consistent with the hypothesis that fluoxetine (Prozac®) is effective in reducing pain severity and the distress and interference associated with pain. The results also suggest that the addition of CBT improves the patients' control over their lives. None

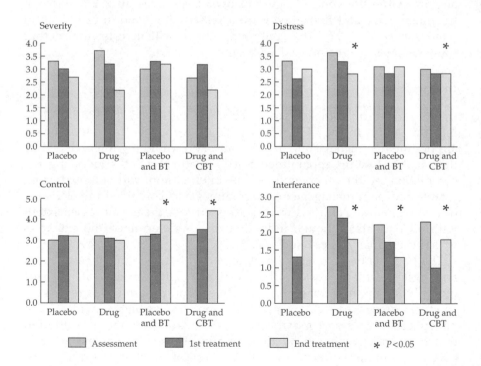

Fig. 6.1 Median multidimensional pain inventory (MPI) scores of patients in the EFP project.

of the patients had initial scores that would indicate clinical depression, so the pain relief appears to be independent of any antidepressant effect.

The dropout was highest in the CBT group and may reflect a difficulty in time commitments. Pilowsky *et al.* (1995) have suggested that patients find CBT more demanding, and feel threatened by the psychological nature of treatment. It is important therefore that patients are assessed for psychological suitability for treatment. Walker (1998) has suggested that the design of clinical trials for conditions involving unexplained symptoms should take into account depression, childhood maltreatment status, and chronic and social stressors. In a further study comparing hypnosis and relaxation, but using briefer CBT techniques, there was less dropout but equal improvement, suggesting that the patients may have found it more acceptable. CBT undoubtedly has a role in chronic idiopathic facial pain, but patients must be assessed before treatment and patient choice of treatment must be taken seriously.

CONCLUSION

The use of CBT in the management of chronic idiopathic facial pain is in the early stages of development. Many of the issues faced by these patients are appropriate for CBT management. Early outcome data suggest that it is a valuable treatment for this distressing condition. The role of CBT in facial pain continues to be investigated. It may be that the demanding nature of CBT requires that it is adapted for a facial pain population.

REFERENCES

Beck, A. T. (1967). *Cognitive therapy and the emotional disorders*. International Universities Press, New York.

Dworkin, S. F., Turner, J. A., Wilson, L., *et al.* (1994). Brief cognitive behaviour intervention for temporomandibular disorders. *Pain*, **59**, 175–87.

Gamsa, A. (1994). The role of psychological factors in chronic pain. I: A half-century study. II: A critical appraisal. *Pain*, **57**, 5–29.

Glasgow, R. E., Hollis, J. F., McRae, S. G., Lando, H. A., and LaChance, P. (1991). Providing an integrated programme of low intensity tobacco cessation services in a health maintenance organisation. *Health Education Research*, **6**, 87–99.

Guthrie, E. (1995). Treatment of functional somatic symptoms: psychodynamic treatment. In R. Mayou, C. Bass and M. Sharpe (Eds). *Treatment of functional somatic symptoms*, pp. 144–60. Oxford University Press, Oxford.

Guthrie, E. and Creed, F. H. (1991). A controlled trial of psychological treatment for irritable bowel. *Gastroenterology*, **100**, 450–7.

Harrison, S. *et al.* (1997). A comparison of antidepressant medication alone and in conjunction with cognitive behaviour therapy for chronic idiopathic facial pain. Proceedings of the Eighth World Congress on pain. (ed. T. Jesson and J. A. Turner), pp. 663–672. IASP Press, Seattle.

Hawton, K. E., Salkovskis, P. M., Kirk, J., and Clark, D. M. (1989). *Cognitive behaviour therapy for psychiatric problems: a practical guide.* Oxford Medical Publishers, Oxford.

Hazard, R. G., Benedix, A. and Genwich, J. W. (1991). Disability exaggeration as a predictor of functional restoration outcome for patients with chronic low back pain. *Spine,* **16,** 295–306.

Holroyd, K. A., Nash, J. M., Pingle, J. D., Cordingly, G. E., and Jerome, A. (1991). A comparison of pharmacological (amitriptyline HCL) and nonpharmacological (cognitive behavioural) therapies for chronic tension headaches. *Journal of Consulting and Clinical Psychology,* **59,** 121–33.

Kerns, R. D., Turk, D. C., Holzman, A. D., and Rudy, T. E. (1986). The efficacy of a cognitive behavioural group approach for the treatment of chronic pain. *Clinical Journal of Pain,* **2,** 195–203.

Klepac, R. C., Klauge, G., Dowling, J., and McDonald, M. (1981). Direct and generalised components of stress inoculation for increased pain tolerance. *Behaviour Therapy,* **12,** 417–27.

Klimes, I., Mayou, R. A., Pearce, M. J., and Fagg, J. R. (1990). Psychological treatment for atypical non-cardiac chest pain: a controlled evaluation. *Psychological medicine,* **20,** 605–11.

Manchini, V. S., Peterson, R. A., and Maruta, T. (1998). Changes in perception of illness and psychosocial adjustment—findings of a pain management program. *Clinical Journal of Pain,* **4,** 249–56.

Nicholas, M. K., Wilson, P. H., and Goyen, J. (1992). Comparison of a cognitive behavioural group treatment and an alternative non-psychological treatment for chronic low back pain. *Pain,* **48,** 339–47.

O'Leary, A., Shor, S., Lorig, K., and Holman, H. R. (1988). A cognitive–behavioural treatment for rheumatoid arthritis. *Health Psychology,* **7,** 527–44.

Olson, R. E. and Malow, R. M. (1987). Effects of biofeedback and psychotherapy on patients with myofacial pain dysfunction who are nonresponsive to conventional treatments. *Rehabilitation Psychology,* **32,** 195–205.

Pilowsky, I., Spence, N., Rouncefell, B., Forsten, C., and Soda, J. (1995). Outpatient cognitive behavioural therapy with amitriptyline for chronic non-malignant pain: a comparative study with 6 months follow up. *Pain,* **60,** 49–54.

Salkovskis, P. M. (1989). Somatic problems. In K. Hawton, P. M. Salkovskis, J. Kirk and D. M. Clarke (Eds). *Cognitive behaviour therapy for psychiatric problems: a practical guide,* pp. 235–76. Oxford Medical Publishers, Oxford.

Sharpe, M., Hawton, K., Simkin, S., Surawy, C., Hackman, A., Klimes, I., Peto, R., Warrell, D., and Seagroatt, V. (1996). Cognitive behaviour therapy for the chronic fatigue syndrome: a randomised controlled trial. *British Medical Journal,* **312,** 22–6.

Skinner, J. B., Erkine, A., Pearce, S., Rubenstein, I. , Taylor, M., and Foster, C. (1990). The evaluation of a cognitive behavioural treatment programme in outpatients with chronic pain. *Journal of Psychosomatic Research,* **34,** 13–19.

Speckens, A. E. M., van Hemert, A. M., Spinhoven, P., Hawton, K. E., Bolk, J. H., and Rooijmans, H. G. M. (1995). Cognitive behaviour therapy for medically unexplained physical symptoms: a randomised controlled trial. *British Medical Journal*, **311**, 1328–32.

Spence, S. H. (1989). Cognitive behaviour therapy in the management of chronic, occupational pain of the upper limbs. *Behaviour Research and Therapy*, **27**, 435–46.

Tota-Faucette, M. E., Gil, K. M., Williams, D. A., Feeke, F. J., and Goli, V. (1993). Predictors of response to pain management treatment. *Clinical Journal of Pain*, **9**, 115–23.

Turk, D. C. and Meichenbaum, D. (1995). A cognitive behavioural approach to pain management. In: Textbook of pain, (ed. R. Wall and P. D. Melzack), pp. 1337–48. Churchill Livingstone, London.

Turk, D. C. and Rudy, T. E. (1990). Neglected factors in chronic pain treatment outcome studies—referral patterns, failure to attend treatment and attrition. *Pain*, **43**, 7–25.

Turner, J. A. and Chapman, C. R. (1982). Psychological interventions for chronic pain: a critical self review. II: Operant conditioning, hypnosis and cognitive behavioural therapy. *Pain*, **12**, 23–46.

Turner, J. A. and Clancy, S. L. (1988). Comparison of operant behavioural and cognitive behavioural group treatment for chronic low back pain. *Journal of Consulting and Clinical Psychology*, **56**, 261–6.

Walker, I. (1998). Designing clinical trials for the treatment of medically unexplained physical symptoms. *Journal of Psychosomatic Research*, **44**, 197–207.

Williams, C. de C. and Erskine, A. (1995). Chronic pain. In *Health psychology: processes and applications*, (2nd edn), (ed. A. Broome and S. Llewelyn). Chapman & Hall, London.

7

Disorders of appearance

Susan J. Cunningham, Charlotte Feinmann, and Richard Ibbetson

INTRODUCTION

Beauty is in the eye of the beholder.

This well-known statement reinforces how difficult it is to measure facial aesthetics objectively. The concepts of beauty and facial attractiveness have altered throughout history but are the source of much debate even today. There is no 'ideal'. Perceptions of facial attractiveness vary from person to person and also vary depending on the 'norm' for that particular population. The physical attractiveness stereotype is likely to remain the subject of many more research studies.

THE IMPORTANCE OF FACIAL ATTRACTIVENESS

Beauty is a greater recommendation than any letter of introduction.
(Aristotle's dictum)

Physical attractiveness is a legitimate and very important psychological variable in the field of appearance. A person's physical appearance is the characteristic which is most obvious to others in social interactions, and attractive people are frequently perceived as being more friendly, sensitive, and successful than those who are unattractive (Dion *et al.* 1972).

There is a great deal of evidence to suggest that unattractive individuals are discriminated against in a wide range of situations and that there exist stereotyped notions of the personality traits possessed by individuals of varying attractiveness. This 'discrimination' starts early in life. Teachers, rating unfamiliar children on the basis of photographs and identical record cards, believed attractive children to be more popular with their peers, more intelligent, and more likely to have successful academic careers (Clifford and Walster 1973). A study by Dion *et al.* (1972) in which college students assessed photographs and then answered questions about the subjects, found that attractive individuals were perceived to possess more socially desirable personalities, to be more likely to secure prestigious jobs and to find a partner and marry early. Thus supporting the 'what is beautiful is good' theory.

Therefore, the assumption must be that physical attractiveness functions as an elicitor of differential behaviour, with attractive individuals receiving more favourable social exchanges than unattractive persons. An increasing number of researchers believe that there is an important association between outer physical appearance and inner behavioural processes. As long ago as 1974, Berscheid and Walster proposed a potential relationship between perceptions of an individual's physical attractiveness, the behaviour towards that person, and the development of certain social characteristics by them. This may go some way to explaining the situation in which individuals with a facial handicap frequently complain they are rejected by others and that people behave in a negative manner in social situations (Bull and Stevens 1981; Rumsey *et al.* 1982). Rumsey *et al.* (1982) showed that although people do behave in a negative manner, facially disfigured individuals often exhibit shyness and defensiveness. This behaviour of those with facial deformities is, in part, a response to the negative behaviour towards them in many social situations.

The profound significance of the face and also society's prejudice against anyone with an atypical appearance means that a facial deformity may be a severe handicap in a wide range of different situations.

DENTOFACIAL DEFORMITY AND ORTHODONTIC TREATMENT

The oral region plays an important role in determining overall facial attractiveness and certain oral features are known to be associated with particular characteristics (for example, a class III malocclusion may be perceived as aggressive, or a class II as weak or stupid). A study by Shaw *et al.* (1980) investigated the extent to which dental deformities in children evoked teasing and ridicule. They found that a number of children were teased about their dental characteristics and admitted to being upset by it. This tendency for dentofacial features to be the cause of teasing was reinforced further in the second part of the same study when children were asked to describe faces and give the person a nickname. In a large number of cases a name was given which related to the dental features.

In another study using facial photographs, Shaw (1981) found that children with a normal dental appearance were judged by both peers and lay adults as being more attractive, more desirable as a friend, and less likely to behave in an aggressive manner than identical faces with dental anomalies. However, background attractiveness of the face was of greater importance than the dental appearance.

Presentation and management

Interest in dental health and dental aesthetics has increased dramatically over the past two or three decades. Along with this, the demand for orthodontic treatment has increased enormously in both adult and child populations. The functional and psychological benefits of orthodontic treatment remain uncertain. Very few malocclusions can be classified as being seriously handicapping, and much of orthodontic treatment is aimed at cosmetic improvement with the aim of enhancing the patient's perception of their own appearance and, hopefully, enhancing their self-esteem. To the majority of patients, the psychological benefits of treatment prevail over improvements in function and in dental health. This in itself is influenced by the aesthetic norms for that particular society and, in addition, everyone has their own personal norms.

Espeland and Stenvik (1991) described three types of response to self dental appearance:

- Persons with a near ideal occlusion or only minor discrepancies who appreciate their good dentofacial appearance.
- Those individuals who accept moderate deviations from the ideal. This group may be divided into two: those who perceive the deviations accurately but are prepared to accept them, and those who are not able to identify the deviations.
- Those persons who do not find moderate deviations from the ideal acceptable and relate their dissatisfaction to these traits.

These three types of response explain why an orthodontist may see some patients with marked deviations who are quite happy with their appearance and yet others demand treatment for very minor discrepancies which would be perfectly acceptable to the majority of the population. The latter group requires very careful management and it must be explained that if treatment is carried out, the net benefit will be small and that there is also relapse potential. If a decision is made to provide treatment, careful documentation of all discussions and completion of a consent form should ensure that both clinician and patient fully understand the situation.

Patients with a dentofacial anomaly may be at a disadvantage for two reasons: their self-esteem and self-confidence may be adversely affected, and the anomaly may cause undesirable responses such as teasing and name-calling. Therefore, demand for orthodontic treatment for aesthetic reasons may not be just vanity but may be a valid intuition of social response. Kerosuo *et al.* (1995) studied the influence of incisal malocclusion on the social attractiveness of young adults by asking students to rank photographs on a variety of characteristics. They found that visible anterior malocclusions, such as crowding or a diastema, had a detrimental effect on perceived social success (for example, beauty, intelligence, and social class). However, dental and facial attractiveness did not influence human virtues such as goodness or honesty. In fact, there was a tendency for the more unattractive appearance to evoke more generous judgements concerning these traits.

Controversy remains regarding the psychological effects of malocclusions and also the effect of treatment on body image and self-concept. It is frequently assumed that adolescents with a malocclusion must possess negative self-esteem and that treatment must improve it. Albino *et al.* (1994) found that parent-, peer-, and self-evaluations of dentofacial attractiveness significantly improved after treatment, but there was no evidence that treatment improved parental and self-evaluations of social competency and self-esteem. Similar findings were reported by O'Regan *et al.* (1991), who noted that an improvement in dental aesthetics does not necessarily imply any increase in self-esteem. However, it is difficult to believe that improvements in dentofacial attractiveness following treatment have no effect on self-concept in a society that values facial attractiveness so highly.

It is likely that general dental practitioners and orthodontists are far more critical of dentofacial aesthetics than are the general public (Prahl-Andersen *et al.* 1979; Kerr and O'Donnell 1990; Cochrane *et al.* 1997). It is therefore important that treatment is not forced on those patients who do not perceive a problem, as it is likely to result in failed co-operation.

The perceived need for treatment by the child and their parents still plays a persuasive element in the allocation of resources, but with the constraints currently being placed as a result of lack of funding, this may not have quite the same impact as in the past. In a number of cases, children are treated because this is what the parent wants and not because the child desires treatment. To some extent this is understandable, but caution must be used in those cases where the parent is very much more motivated than the child.

Orthodontics has traditionally been a speciality devoted to children and adolescents, and only recently has there been an increased demand for adult orthodontics, particularly in the UK. As a result of this, there are few studies investigating adult patients who have undergone conventional orthodontics, although there are many studies involving adults who have undergone orthodontics in conjunction with orthognathic surgery. Varela and Garcia-Camba (1995) studied 40 adults with moderate to severe malocclusions who were treated orthodontically. They found that although overall and facial body image improved following treatment, self-esteem did not change over time. They also found that the psychological profile of adults electing to undergo conventional orthodontics was basically normal. These results compare well with other studies investigating patients undergoing orthognathic surgery (Peterson and Topazian 1976; Kiyak *et al.* 1982*a*; Flanary *et al.* 1990).

As with adolescent patients, the prime motivating factor for adults seeking orthodontic treatment is aesthetics. However, the clinician must be particularly alert to those patients who may pose problems with respect to their expectations from treatment. Patients displaying these characteristics may benefit from psychiatric counselling prior to commencing treatment so that all involved in the treatment are aware of what the patient expects. This group of patients must be made fully aware of all aspects of treatment, such as length of treatment, type of retention proposed, and any problems that may be anticipated.

DENTOFACIAL DEFORMITY AND RESTORATIVE TREATMENT

Patients who are seeking restorative treatment to improve their appearance seem to be similar to those pursuing orthodontic treatment. However, it is apparent that dentists' perceptions of what the aesthetic priorities might be are not generally the same as those of the patient. Neumann *et al.* (1989) indicated that aspects of dental appearance were not ranked in the same order by patients and dentists. Furthermore, dentists tend to recommend treatment on the basis of their own experience rather than on the wishes of the patient (Brisman 1980; Goldstein and Lancaster 1984). There is no 'correct' list of aesthetic priorities and it is therefore incumbent on the dentist to seek the views of patients as to what they like or dislike, rather than relying on their own judgement. The dentist must facilitate the process of allowing patients to describe what they wish rather then directing the process.

If dissatisfaction with restorative dental treatment is to be avoided, the initial assessment of the individual must be considered and effective. The patient must be asked very specifically to define the problems that they wish to be addressed. The dentist needs to be certain that these wishes can be met, and must explain and demonstrate the limitations of what can be achieved. The dentist should also be alert to the patient who seems to have complaints that are out of proportion to the dentist's perception of the problem, or who describes their presenting problem in a level of detail that seems inappropriate given the nature of the aesthetic defect. Such patients very often give a history of previous failed treatment: if the latter is the case, the dentist may be well advised to contact the previous practitioner.

Post-treatment dissatisfaction can best be avoided by careful planning and involvement of the patient in decision making. Where changes in appearance are planned, it is essential that a patient be shown a 'mock-up' of the final result. This can be discussed with the patient and it may also be helpful for it to be taken home by the patient where it can be examined more carefully and discussed with friends or family. Furthermore, patients' expectations should not be raised to the point where disappointment is likely. The value of clear explanations, taking time with the patient, and developing the professional relationship are important to patient satisfaction (Oates *et al.* 1995).

All restorative dental care is founded on the establishment of health of the tissues and the elimination of active dental disease. This provides an opportunity to assess the patient's response to this initial treatment and to continue to assess their presenting complaint and its appropriateness in more detail.

ORTHOGNATHIC SURGERY

Orthognathic surgery has evolved over a number of years to correct facial and dental abnormalities which exist as a result of skeletal disproportion and are therefore out of the scope of routine orthodontic treatment. Orthognathic surgery has assumed an important role in both orthodontics and maxillofacial surgery over the past three decades. It is likely that the 'legitimization' of cosmetic-type surgery has increased the demand for treatment even further. The ultimate treatment plan is based not only on the clinician's assessment of aesthetics, function, and stability, but also on the patient's perceptions of what he wishes to obtain from treatment (Kiyak *et al.* 1985). Patients often perceive their own facial profiles quite differently to clinicians and this reinforces the need for good communication when explaining surgical procedures (Bell *et al.* 1985).

Presentation

Orthognathic treatment is undertaken for aesthetic and/or functional reasons. A desire for aesthetic improvement has been cited as a major motivating factor for those undergoing treatment (Wictorin *et al.* 1969; Kiyak *et al.* 1981; Jacobson 1984; Flanary *et al.* 1985; Finlay *et al.* 1995).

It has been assumed in the past that women place greater importance on physical attractiveness than men (Kurtz 1969) and that women seeking cosmetic procedures are more difficult to satisfy than men. It may be anticipated, however, that men and women today pay equal attention to physical attractiveness, and that society's acceptance of males seeking cosmetic surgery has led to an increase in the number of males seeking aesthetic treatment. Kiyak *et al.* (1981) studied personality, motives, and surgical outcome in men and women undergoing orthognathic treatment. Self-ratings of body image were within the normal range for both males and females and although sex differences emerged in the motives for surgery, these were not significant. There were no significant sex differences in any of the satisfaction variables post-surgery and males and females were equally satisfied with the results.

Initial assessment

The initial assessment of an orthognathic patient is one of the most critical stages in treatment. It may require several visits in order to ascertain the patient's main problems and the changes he desires. Following this, the clinician must decide whether these expectations can be met with treatment. The source of motivation is one of the crucial factors to be established—two types of motivation have been described (Edgerton and Knorr 1971):

1.   External: these patients seek treatment in order to please others, e.g. a parent or spouse, or because they think that surgery will please others and make their external environment easier. These patients require careful psychological assessment and counselling prior to any treatment. Surgery is unlikely to achieve what they want, instead a change in the external environment is needed.

2.   Internal: these individuals usually have long-standing inner feelings about deficiencies in their appearance and feel that their appearance blocks their enjoyment of life. They usually make better surgical candidates; however, they still require careful assessment.

The ability to identify those patients who would make inappropriate surgical candidates does not appear to exist as yet. However, there are several characteristics that should make the clinician wary. Some of these will be discussed in a later section covering body dysmorphic disorder but there are others which are perhaps more subtle indicators. Edgerton and Knorr (1971) and Peterson and Topazian (1976) described some of the characteristics that may influence the patient's response to treatment:

* Those patients who have developed a good 'body image' despite their facial deformity are thought to make more appropriate surgical candidates.

* Those individuals who can give positive answers to the questions 'What do you think is wrong?', 'Why do you want treatment?', 'Why

have you decided to seek treatment now?', and 'What do you expect from surgery?' are likely to be better candidates than those with vague answers. A vague response is a worrying sign and further counselling should be considered. It may be that the patient is not able to verbalize what he wants from treatment and that this can be ascertained by careful questioning; however, it may be that the patient really does not have any idea what he expects from treatment.

- Patients with a long history of unhappiness about a particular feature are usually better patients that those who have only just decided they want treatment. The latter group may have decided they have a problem as a response to a major life event such as divorce or a death in the family, and this group of patients needs to be assessed very carefully before agreeing to any treatment.

- Care should also be taken with those who want secondary gain from treatment (for example, a better job, a new relationship), those who are seeking treatment to please someone else, and those who have 'subjective deformities' which are minimal and would be tolerated by the majority of individuals.

Psychological evaluation of patients is recognized as being difficult, but the success of surgery may well depend on careful patient assessment and selection. Those patients who the clinician feels concerned about should be referred to a psychologist or liaison psychiatrist for more thorough assessment before proceeding further. A delay in starting treatment will give adequate time for this assessment and will also determine how keen the patient is to have surgery.

Satisfaction and dissatisfaction

The lack of standardized outcome measures in the field of orthognathic treatment means that patient satisfaction and dissatisfaction have become traditional methods of postoperative evaluation (Hutton 1967; Crowell et al. 1970; Kiyak et al. 1981, 1984, 1986; Jacobson 1984; Flanary et al. 1990; Finlay et al. 1995; Cunningham et al. 1996). Fortunately, the majority of patients are satisfied with the outcome of orthognathic treatment. Flanary et al. (1985) reviewed the literature and found that between 92 and 100 per cent of patients were happy with the results of treatment. This high rate of satisfaction contrasts with some studies involving cosmetic surgery (cosmetic surgery in this context includes rhinoplasty, breast augmentation, breast reduction). Postoperative problems appear to be less frequent in orthognathic patients (Heldt et al. 1982). Several reasons have been proposed as to why this should be so: Edgerton and Knorr (1971) suggested that orthognathic patients receive more support from friends and family because they believe the surgery is being carried out for both aesthetic and functional reasons, and this is somehow considered more legitimate than treatment solely for cosmetic reasons. This may apply less now that cosmetic surgery is more 'socially acceptable'. Orthognathic patients are often referred for treatment rather than initiating the referral themselves, and this may also be a factor in selecting a psychologically different population (Jensen 1978). In addition, the majority of orthognathic patients are in their late teens and early twenties and may adjust more readily than mature adults (Heldt *et al.* 1982).

Hutton (1967) was one of the first clinicians to study postoperative satisfaction in the field of orthognathic treatment. His retrospective study assessed 32 patients who had undergone surgery to correct prognathism and found that all but one patient were pleased with the change in their appearance. The majority of patients also reported increased self-confidence and fewer fears in social interactions. A number of studies followed this (Wictorin *et al.* 1969; Crowell *et al.* 1970; Hillerström *et al.* 1971, Laufer *et al.* 1976; Olson and Laskin 1980), but it was not until the 1980s that the results of a longitudinal study undertaken by Kiyak and colleagues at the University of Washington, Seattle were published. The data from this study showed high levels of satisfaction postoperatively.

Kiyak *et al.* (1982*a*) found that those patients who experienced less pain and numbness than expected were more satisfied and experienced higher self-esteem than those who experienced as much, or more, pain and numbness than expected. This reinforces the need to inform patients of all possible problems they may encounter if maximum satisfaction is to be achieved.

Satisfaction with surgery, self-esteem, and body image reached peak levels at 4 months post-surgery and then declined at the 9-month stage (Kiyak *et al.* 1982*b*). In some cases this may have been due to continued orthodontic treatment, and reinforces the need for only a relatively short period of postoperative orthodontics. In other cases, patients may have expected greater changes in their life as a whole and at 9 months realized that these were not realistic expectations.

A later study (Kiyak *et al.* 1984) showed that if patients perceived aesthetic improvements, their satisfaction was high regardless of functional problems such as paraesthesia or TMJ clicks. This paper also stressed that the psychological upheaval experienced around the time of surgery continues for a considerable time afterwards, and continued contact between patient and clinician should be maintained until this period of trauma is over—this may be as long as 2 years after surgery for some individuals.

Orthognathic treatment has traditionally been viewed as treatment undergone by patients in their late teens and early twenties. Ostler and Kiyak (1991) showed a high level of satisfaction in all age groups. Age did not appear to be a major factor in outcome and satisfaction, which suggests that not only the younger age groups benefit from this type of surgery. However, older patients may require more support in the postoperative period in adapting to their new appearance.

Although the majority of patients are satisfied with the outcomes of treatment, there are some cases of postoperative dissatisfaction. In the majority of cases this is due to an unfavourable interpersonal relationship between clinician and patient rather than due to the technical skills of the clinician. Dissatisfaction with surgical outcome may manifest itself in a number of different ways, including psychological disturbance, postoperative depression, interpersonal problems, and seeking additional surgical procedures.

Macgregor (1981) attributed dissatisfaction following apparently successful surgery to one of the following groups of factors:

- Patient factors: unrealistic expectations; serious psychological problems; patient had surgery on impulse or to please someone else.

- Clinician factors: hasty evaluation of the patient; failure to prepare the patient adequately; minimizing what is involved; not listening to postoperative problems.

- Clinician–patient interaction: poor communication; personality conflict.

Avoiding dissatisfaction and dealing with problems

Postsurgical dissatisfaction can best be avoided by careful patient assessment initially and by thorough explanation of all the problems which may be expected during treatment and also in the postoperative phase. This information should be given verbally but should also be supported with information leaflets. Most patients will remember only a small percentage of what they are told in a clinical situation, especially if they are nervous, and this needs to be supplemented (Flanary and Alexander 1983; Rittersma 1989; Cunningham *et al.* 1996).

The importance of family and friends in the postoperative phase can not be over emphasized, and friends and relatives should be encouraged to attend certain key appointments during the treatment. Holman *et al.* (1995) found that the availability of support, and satisfaction with support from specific members of the patient's support group were significantly associated with satisfaction in the early post-surgery phase. Reich (1975) reported 100 consecutive rhinoplasty patients. All patients were assessed as having normal personalities and realistic expectations preoperatively but postoperatively 24 expressed dissatisfaction. All 24 said that a close friend or contact had either failed to notice a change in their appearance or had made some disparaging remark or pointed out an irregularity. Therefore, the reactions of others during the post-treatment period are important in the process of integrating their new appearance into their body image and self-esteem.

A patient's dissatisfaction with treatment will not always present in a straightforward manner. Dissatisfaction may be resolved in one of several directions, such as attention-seeking devices, requests for further surgery, or litigation (Reich 1975). It is important that the clinician is vigilant and should any of these occur in the postoperative phase, he should be aware that it may be a result of dissatisfaction with outcome. In the early postoperative stages, this may be due to the psychological upheaval which the patient is experiencing and he may require simple reassurance that the situation will improve. Other patients may experience negative feelings due to continued orthodontic treatment (Kiyak *et al.* 1982*a*, 1984, 1986) and, if possible, orthodontic treatment should be kept to a minimum following surgery. In a small number of cases, the problem will be less easy to resolve and sensitive management by an experienced clinician is called for.

Depression is not uncommon following orthognathic surgery and may manifest itself as poor appetite or weight loss, insomnia or hyper-somnia, loss of energy, feelings of worthlessness, inability to concentrate, or suicidal thoughts (Stewart and Sexton 1987). Patients and families should be warned that a short period of depression is likely and this will then reduce the impact of the problem should it occur. Any patient who shows signs of depression postoperatively should be taken seriously and offered treatment. It is important that treatment should be available immediately and that patients do not have to wait long periods to see someone experienced in the management of these problems. Sometimes a short course of antidepressants will produce marked improvements, in other cases more prolonged treatment may be required.

CLEFT PALATE AND CRANIOFACIAL PATIENTS

Much of the research in this area has centred on the psychological problems faced by patients with clefts of the lip and/or palate. Fewer studies have looked at those individuals with other craniofacial deformities.

It is easy to assume that the more severe a facial deformity is, the more severe the psychological effects will be. Macgregor (1970) and Reich (1969) were the first to notice that this did not necessarily seem to be the case. Reich (1969) proposed that this was due to the fact that severely deformed individuals can confidently predict a negative response, whereas those with milder abnormalities are never quite sure what response they will encounter—whether it will be pity, ridicule, or if they will be completely ignored. Lansdown *et al.* (1991) found that there was a trend for mildly deformed individuals to have the lowest self-concept, but this did not reach statistically significant levels.

Those who support reconstruction in early childhood believe that normalization of craniofacial features prior to the individual developing a sense of deformity yields positive psychological benefits (Lefebvre and Munro 1978). Barden *et al.* (1988) stated that the major rationales for craniofacial surgery include:

- an improvement in the patient's physical appearance;
- improvements in appearance will then elicit more favourable social reactions and interactions;
- improvements in social reactions and interactions will enhance the psychological adjustment of the patient.

Their study (Barden *et al.* 1988) involved showing pre- and post-surgery photographs of patients with a wide range of craniofacial malformations to a rating panel and asking them to predict their response to the individual in that picture. Observers predicted more positive responses to the patients in the photographs taken following surgery than to the same individuals prior to surgery. If such treatment at least partly counteracts these consistent negative responses, then the patients may develop improved social skills and feel more confident in social interactions.

Psychosocial effects

Barden *et al.* (1989) studied the effect of craniofacial deformity on the quality of mother–infant interactions, and although mothers of facially deformed infants rated their parental satisfaction more positively than did mothers of normal infants, they behaved in a consistently less nurturant manner than mothers of non-deformed children. This may influence future psychological development of the infant. Those children who have a positive family background are more likely to develop higher self-esteem than those who constantly experience negative feedback (Clifford and Crocker 1971; Palkes *et al.* 1986).

Studies of cleft-palate individuals have frequently found that the differences on psychosocial variables between those with clefts and control populations are small and inconsistent. Brantley and Clifford (1979) proposed that a cleft adolescent should be classified as a normal subject rather than a member of a 'unique group'. This hypothesis was upheld by Clifford *et al.* (1972) who found that adults with cleft lip and palate had a relatively high level of satisfaction with their bodies and themselves, and tended to perceive low influence of the cleft on education, dating, etc.

Other studies present opposing views. Harper and Richman (1978), in their study of cleft children and children with orthopaedic impairment, found that cleft adolescents showed significantly greater stress and discomfort relating to interpersonal relationships. Kapp (1979) also noted the negative effects of clefts: cleft children reported significantly greater unhappiness than non-cleft children and also expressed greater dissatisfaction with personal appearance. Cleft females reported highest levels of unhappiness and dissatisfaction. It may be that females are more affected by their disability because of the importance of physical attractiveness in today's society. Peter and Chinsky (1974a, b) and Peter *et al.* (1975) found no significant differences between cleft and non-cleft groups with respect to educational attainment, but cleft subjects appeared to experience some limitations in their ability to secure vocational and economic rewards from society. In addition, they found that those with clefts married at a significantly lower rate when compared with siblings and that there was a substantial delay in the timing of their first marriage.

Management of psychosocial problems

Research efforts in this area must be directed towards the expansion of multidisciplinary teams which include a psychologist, psychiatrist, or other mental health professional trained in the special needs of facially deformed individuals (Broder and Richman 1987).

These children and their families face both social and psychological stresses which can negatively affect their quality of life. Because there is no way of predicting which patients will develop problems, counselling should be widely available throughout treatment. Families may also require the support of the mental health professional, particularly at important stages of treatment, such as prior to major surgery.

In some cases, benefit may be obtained by teaching social skills in order to improve communication and make the patient more acceptable to his peer group (Kapp-Simon 1995). The development of psychotherapy programmes may also fulfil a useful role. In order to do this effectively, more longitudinal studies are required to determine how the social environment of the cleft child differs from that of the non-cleft child, and to study the basis for individual differences (Bennett and Stanton 1993).

A significant number of individuals recognize their own social adjustment problems. Self-reported problems are indicative of the need for psychological assessment and possibly intervention (Richman 1983).

FACIAL DEFORMITY AS A RESULT OF SURGICAL INTERVENTION FOR HEAD AND NECK CANCER

Many cancer patients will experience psychosocial problems both during and after their treatment. These may range from anxiety and depression to body-image concerns and increased stress within the family unit. Patients who experience disfiguring surgery for head and neck cancer may be particularly vulnerable to a breakdown in communication with a spouse or other family members (Esterling 1996). Most of the functions associated with human interaction are centred around the head. It is, therefore, not surprising that to face a dramatic change in facial form and function is devastating to those patients who undergo surgery for head and neck cancers (David and Barritt 1982). The voice and facial appearance also comprise major aspects of self-concept which develops throughout life from as early as infancy. Self-concept is influenced by the development of the body itself and also by cognitive function, perceptions of body stimuli, comparison with others, and the perceived reactions of others (Shapiro and Kornfeld 1987). Changes in body image occur in a complex manner following the dramatic changes imposed by the surgery, and these changes are affected by social and psychological factors as well as by the physical changes.

Loss of facial function and form has massive implications to both the patient and his family. Relatively few patients fail to adapt psychologically to their new appearance, but most will experience staring and possibly hurtful comments which call for tolerance on their behalf (Olson and Shedd 1978). Although the majority do adapt to their change in facial appearance, almost all will require a great deal of support, both from professionals and from their family and friends. West (1977) found that 86 per cent of patients who underwent surgery for head and neck cancer adapted to the facial deformity and proposed that the driving forces during the adaptive phase included maintaining self-esteem and a positive self-concept, acceptance by family and hospital staff, a perceived lessening of the importance of attractiveness with advancing age, and the nature of the disease itself (for example, the thought that disfigurement is better than death). This study showed the ability of these patients to adapt to their facial deformity in a wide range of situations, including work and social activities.

Managing the surgical patient

The importance of a team approach has the same benefit as in the management of craniofacial patients, and this should exist in the hospital setting as well as in the community setting when the patient returns home (David and Barritt 1982).

All patients should undergo a psychosocial assessment preoperatively, postoperatively, and soon after returning home. The preoperative assessment allows the patient and his family to ask as many questions as they need, and they can also be made aware of the practical support available to them. In addition, those in charge of their care must ascertain the patient's strengths, weaknesses, and his ability to cope in a crisis situation—this will allow postoperative care and support to be planned.

In the immediate postoperative phase, most patients will experience reactive depression, which calls for support from all members of the team as well as from immediate family. This depression is a result of not only the facial deformity but also the problems experienced with speech, eating, and drinking. It is important to distinguish between reactive and endogenous depression as the latter may require medication and psychiatric care.

The problems faced by patients who experienced debilitating facial surgery led to the increased demand to avoid surgery that produces marked facial deformity and to use flaps which leave less visible scarring. The ability to reconstruct defects during surgery, or by the provision of prosthetic devices if surgical reconstruction is not possible, ensures that patients can start adapting to their change in appearance early in the postoperative phase.

It is common for patients to feel anxious about leaving hospital with an altered facial appearance, and relatives and friends must be counselled in order to understand and support the disfigured patient. Loss of body image and self-worth require considerable effort to restore. In some cases, group treatment programmes may be useful in allowing the patient to realize that he is not the only individual with that problem, and other patients may also be able to offer practical advice and support.

Esterling (1996) proposed that one way of avoiding some of the problems associated with the effects of the cancer and the associated treatment is for the patient to exert control over them. He described four types of control that may help the patient to reduce the associated stress:

(1) behavioural control: a belief that you can affect the associated problems by direct action;

(2) cognitive action: the ability to affect the negative aspects of the illness and treatment by thinking about it differently or from other perspectives;

(3) information control: if the individuals have received information about the events, they are more likely to have feelings of control;

(4) retrospective control: this involves making attributions about the cause of the past events.

Which form of psychosocial intervention is most useful will depend on the type of illness and also the problems that the individual is facing. However, they all share a common goal and that is to reduce patient distress and to improve quality of life. Esterling (1996) discusses the benefits of patient education and support-group therapy, as well as the use of cognitive behavioural therapy (CBT) which aims to help patients develop a 'fighting spirit' by using the appropriate coping skills and behavioural strategies.

THE PSYCHOLOGICAL IMPACT OF TRAUMATICALLY ACQUIRED FACIAL DEFORMITY

The majority of facial injuries acquired through trauma are as a result of assault or accidents such as motor vehicle crashes. The trend in facial injuries has altered over the past 20 years as a result of seat-belt legislation and tougher drink–driving laws (Magennis *et al.* 1998). The number of facial injuries sustained in road-traffic accidents continues to fall and the number sustained in assaults continues to rise. A recent study in the UK reported 6114 facial injuries in 163 Accident and Emergency Departments over a 1-week period (Hutchison *et al.* 1998). The majority of these injuries were in young males and many were related to excess alcohol consumption.

The term post-traumatic stress disorder (PTSD) was first described in the psychiatric literature in 1980 (American Psychiatric Association 1980) and is associated with nightmares, flashbacks to the traumatic incident, and avoidance of thoughts or reminders of the incident. Mayou *et al.* (1993) studied patients who were injured in motor accidents and found that 8 per cent were suffering from PTSD 1 year afterwards. Shepherd *et al.* (1990) administered the Hospital Anxiety and Depression (HAD) scale to 122 patients 1 week after sustaining a jaw fracture and found that more than 10 per cent scored higher than 10 on this scale. These scores decreased after 3 months in those individuals who had sustained their injuries in an accident but remained elevated in those who had been assaulted. Bisson *et al.* (1997) administered questionnaires to facial trauma victims at initial assessment and then 7 weeks later. At the follow-up visit, 12 (27 per cent) of patients were diagnosed as suffering from PTSD as defined in DSM-IV (American Psychiatric Association 1994).

Management

It is only relatively recently that the psychological sequelae of facial trauma have been considered. However, recent work suggests that it is not a situation that should be ignored. Facial injuries may result in a whole range of permanent disabilities, ranging from permanent nerve damage to loss of vision (Hutchison *et al.* 1998). If these sequelae are combined with long-lasting psychological problems in a significant number of individuals, then it may be that combined care from both maxillofacial surgeons and psychiatrists or psychologists is required. A review of modes of treatment of PTSD suggests that several approaches are successful, including pharmacological treatment, exposure therapy, and cognitive therapy (Solomon *et al.* 1992). This area requires further investigation in the form of randomized clinical trials.

PSYCHIATRIC DISORDERS OF APPEARANCE: BODY DYSMORPHIC DISORDER

Most clinicians will be familiar with the patient who has a subjective feeling of ugliness or a physical defect that he or she believes is noticeable to others, although the appearance is within normal limits. These situations suggest a diagnosis of dysmorphophobia, which was defined by Morselli as 'the sudden onset and subsequent persistence of an idea of deformity; the individual fears he has become or may become deformed and feels tremendous anxiety of such an awareness' (Morselli 1891).

The term 'dysmorphophobia' has been replaced by the diagnosis 'body dysmorphic disorder' (BDD). The *Diagnostic and Statistical Manual of Mental Disorders IV* (DSM-IV 1994) and ICD-10 (World Health Organization 1992) redefined dysmorphophobia into delusional and non-delusional variants, and the non-delusional variant is now known as BDD. Three criteria must be fulfilled to make a diagnosis of BDD:

1. There is preoccupation with a defect in the appearance. The defect is either imagined, or if a minor defect is present, the individual's concern is excessive.

2. The preoccupation causes significant distress in social, occupational, and other important areas of functioning.

3. The preoccupation is not better accounted for by another mental disorder (for example, anorexia nervosa).

Presenting features and clinical importance

BDD usually begins during adolescence with symptoms persisting over a number of years (Phillips *et al.* 1995) and there is nearly always a delay in seeking treatment (Phillips 1991). The area of concern may remain the same or may change. The imagined defect in appearance frequently affects the head and neck area, which increases the likelihood of the disorder being seen by general dentists, orthodontists, and maxillofacial surgeons. Veale *et al.* (1996) found that 86 per cent of their sample mentioned some aspect of their face. However, any part of the body may be affected and because patients suffering from BDD consult a wide range of specialists, ranging from surgeons to psychiatrists, the demographics are difficult to ascertain.

As a result of the difficulties experienced in reliable data collection, there is conflicting evidence as to the sex bias of the condition. Phillips (1991) quoted a ratio of approximately 1 : 1 female : male; however, Veale *et al.* (1996) found that 75 per cent of their sample was female. This may have been heavily influenced by the fact that some of the patients in their study self-referred following articles in newspapers and in a women's magazine. In contrast, Thomas (1995) found that males outnumbered females in their BDD group.

BDD preoccupations are distressing and time consuming. Patients may spend hours thinking about their defect, studying it in the mirror, or attempting to camouflage the area. This can reach such proportions that they become housebound or even attempt suicide. A study by Phillips *et al.* (1994, cited by Phillips *et al.* 1995) found that 29 per cent of their patients had made suicide attempts and 98 per cent said they had experienced significant impairment in social function. A study by Perugi *et al.* (1997) found that 79 per cent of patients reported excessive mirror checking and 53 per cent reported attempts to camouflage their 'deformity'. As a result of this, almost 90 per cent avoided usual social activities, 52 per cent reported impairment of their academic or job performance, 45 per cent experienced suicidal ideation, and 36 per cent exhibited aggressive behaviour.

BDD patients require careful assessment at initial appointments and it is important that this is by an experienced clinician who does not risk making matters worse by drawing the patient's attention to other potential 'defects'. Referral letters sometimes suggest there is a problem: the referring practitioner may indicate that the patient's worries are over a minor or non-evident problem, or there may have been numerous consultations with other clinicians, all of whom have refused treatment ('doctor shopping'). Frequently the patients are embarrassed by what they perceive to be a dreadful defect and may attempt to hide the problem unless specifically questioned about it. In other cases they will appear intrusive and demand constant reassurance about the supposed defect. They may also attend out-patient clinics with pictures, photographs, or diagrams in an attempt to show that they do have a problem. It is vital that clinicians are aware of the implications in dealing with BDD and are not pushed into inappropriate treatment by persuasive patients.

A study by Thomas and Goldberg (1995) found that a panel of lay judges rated the appearance of the dysmorphophobic group intermediate between that of a control group and a group of patients due to undergo rhinoplasty. The same patients also underwent a procedure called morph-analysis, an accurate method of obtaining facial images. They found that both the rhinoplasty and the dysmorphophobic group deviated from the normal population but not significantly from each other. However, there was little correspondence between the patient's complaint and the actual anomaly in the dysmorphophobic group.

If possible, it is helpful to interview family members. They have often become so used to the problem that they no longer see it as abnormal. It is important that they understand the condition and realize that it is pathological and requires treatment.

It is important to recognize such patients at an early stage if in-appropriate and potentially damaging treatment is to be avoided. The descriptions in the literature of these individuals are so specific that early detection would appear straightforward. This is not the case. The patient affected by BDD may sometimes present with an entirely plausible history and complaint, such that it is not until treatment has begun that the problem becomes apparent. Indeed, patients suffering from BDD may provide a history that encourages intervention: these patients are frequently very well 'educated' dentally. However, the level of detail of their complaint is often not appropriate and it may be that the patient perceives a problem where the dentist does not. A dentist who provides treatment under these circumstances is unlikely to be successful as the treatment inevitably becomes patient-directed.

It might seem surprising that patients suffering from BDD are able to persuade dentists to provide treatment. Frequently, however, their com-plaints and histories do appear plausible initially. This is combined with the fact that in general practice, many dentists practice in isolation from their colleagues, and the majority of the profession who work in practice are not involved in peer review or audit. This makes it difficult to share experiences and knowledge and increases the chances of the patient with BDD being able to persuade the dentist to provide treatment.

Management and treatment options

The management of patients suspected of having BDD depends to some extent on what facilities are available in the area. The three main treatment modalities available are surgery, pharmacological treatment, and counselling and behavioural therapy.

Surgery

(Or other active treatment in the case of the restorative or orthodontic patient.) Patients will frequently pursue surgical treatment for their defect. They may attend numerous surgeons in the hope of finding someone who is willing to operate on them. They may also conceal the fact that they have seen previous clinicians and been refused treatment. Surgery rarely improves the situation and will frequently make it worse, with the patient finding a new 'defect' afterwards (Phillips *et al.* 1995). It is important that clinicians are not pressurized into treating patients against their better judgement, treatment should be provided only where there is clinical justification. There are reports of patients with minimal deformity who have benefited from surgery when treated in conjunction with psychiatric preparation (Reich 1969; Thomas 1984). However, the majority of clinicians support the view that surgery is not helpful in the long term.

Pharmacological treatment

Lack of controlled clinical trials has made the assessment of pharmacological treatment in BDD very difficult. Several reports indicate the effectiveness of antidepressants, particularly selective serotonin reuptake inhibitors (SSRIs). Phillips and co-workers (Phillips and McElroy 1993; Phillips *et al.* 1994) found that both the non-delusional and delusional conditions responded to SSRIs, with a response rate of approximately 60 per cent. Their efficacy, in conjunction with their safety in overdose and low side-effect profile, makes them a popular treatment.

A number of BDD patients also suffer from depression, the two conditions may co-exist or the depression may be secondary to the BDD and its distressing time-consuming behaviour. Phillips *et al.* (1994) found a current prevalence of 59 per cent and a lifetime prevalence of 83 per cent. It seems likely that SSRIs are treating both the BDD and the depression.

Other antidepressants have been shown to be successful in a small number of cases, but the majority have been shown to be largely ineffective. Therefore, although SSRIs are relatively expensive, they are currently the pharmacological agent of choice.

Counselling and behavioural therapy

A number of different treatment options are available, including psychotherapy, systematic desensitization (Munjack 1978), and cognitive behavioural therapy (Rosen *et al.* 1995). Rosen *et al.* (1995) propose a number of different principles used in therapy sessions, including:

- subjects constructing a hierarchy of distressing aspects of their condition and using exposure therapy, thought stopping, and relaxation to stop distress at the sight of the 'defect';

- keeping a body-image diary to record body-image thoughts or beliefs;
- response prevention to reduce checking behaviour.

The authors found that BDD symptoms were significantly reduced in subjects who underwent therapy and the disorder appeared to be eliminated in 82 per cent of cases immediately post-treatment and 77 per cent at follow-up.

CONCLUSIONS

Although recent years have seen a great deal of research in this area, there remains a considerable amount of work to be undertaken in the field of disorders of facial appearance. Certain important concerns such as reasons for dissatisfaction with the results of technically satisfactory surgery, the ability to detect those patients who may be 'inappropriate' for complex treatment, and also the most appropriate methods of providing information are just three of the difficult areas which must be looked at in more detail.

The importance of team care must be emphasized if facially disfigured patients are to obtain the care they require. This can only be achieved through the development of centralized services where all disciplines are represented and a collaborative approach is possible.

REFERENCES

Albino, J. E. N., Lawrence, S. D., and Tedesco, L. A. (1994). Psychological and social effects of orthodontic treatment. *Journal of Behavioral Medicine*, **17**, 81–98.

American Psychiatric Association (1980). *Diagnostic and statistical manual of mental disorders*, (3rd edn). American Psychiatric Press, Washington, DC.

American Psychiatric Association (1994). *Diagnostic and statistical manual of mental disorders*, (4th edn). American Psychiatric Press, Washington, DC.

Barden, R. C., Ford, M. E., Wilhelm, W. M., Rogers-Salyer, M., and Salyer, K. E. (1988). Emotional and behavioural reactions to facially deformed patients before and after craniofacial surgery. *Plastic and Reconstructive Surgery*, **82**, 409–18.

Barden, R. C., Ford, M. E., Jensen, A. G., Rogers-Salyer, M., and Salyer, K. E. (1989). Effects of craniofacial deformity in infancy on the quality of mother–infant interactions. *Child Development*, **60**, 819–24.

Bell, R., Kiyak, H. A., Joondeph, D. R., McNeill, R. W., and Wallen, T. R. (1985). Perceptions of facial profile and their influence on the decision to undergo orthognathic surgery. *American Journal of Orthodontics*, **88**, 323–32.

Bennett, M. E. and Stanton, M. L. (1993). Psychotherapy for persons with craniofacial deformities: can we treat without theory? *Cleft Plate–Craniofacial Journal*, **30**, 406–10.

Berscheid, E. and Walster, E. (1974). Physical attractiveness. In *Advances in experimental social psychology*, (ed. L. Berkowitz), Vol. 6. Academic Press, New York.

Bisson, J. I., Shepherd, J. P., and Dhutia, M. (1997). Psychological sequelae of facial trauma. *Journal of Trauma, Injury, Infection and Critical Care*, **43**, 496–500.

Brantley, H. T. and Clifford, E. (1979). Cognitive, self-concept and body image measures on normal, cleft palate and obese adolescents. *Cleft Plate Journal*, **16**, 177–82.

Brisman, A. S. (1980). Esthetic comparisons of dentists' and patients' concepts. *Journal of the American Dental Association*, **100**, 345–52.

Broder, H. and Richman, L. (1987). An examination of mental health services offered by Cleft/ Craniofacial teams. *Cleft Plate–Craniofacial Journal*, **32**, 104–8.

Bull, R. and Stevens, J. (1981). The effects of facial disfigurement on helping behaviour. *Italian Journal of Psychology*, **8**, 25–33.

Clifford, E. and Crocker, E. (1971). Maternal responses: the birth of a normal child as compared to the birth of a child with a cleft. *Cleft Palate Journal*, **8**, 298–306.

Clifford, E., Crocker, E. C., and Pope, B. A. (1972). Psychological findings in the adulthood of 98 cleft lip–palate children. *Plastic and Reconstructive Surgery*, **50**, 234–7.

Clifford, M. M. and Walster, E. (1973). The effects of physical attractiveness on teacher expectations. *Sociology in Education*, **46**, 248–58.

Cochrane, S. M., Cunningham, S. J., and Hunt, N. P. (1997). Perceptions of facial appearance by orthodontists and the general public. *Journal of Clinical Orthodontics*, **31**, 164–8.

Crowell, N. T., Sazima, H. J., and Elder, S. T. (1970). Survey of patients' attitudes after surgical correction of prognathism. A study of 33 patients. *Journal of Oral Surgery*, **28**, 818–22.

Cunningham, S. J., Hunt, N. P., and Feinmann, C. (1996). Perceptions of outcome following orthognathic surgery. *British Journal of Oral and Maxillofacial Surgery*, **34**, 210–13.

David, D. J. and Barritt, J. A. (1982). Psychosocial implications of surgery for head and neck cancer. *Clinics in Plastic Surgery*, **9**, 327–36.

Dion, K., Berscheid, E., and Walster, E. (1972). What is beautiful is good. *Journal of Personality and Social Psychology*, **24**, 285–90.

Edgerton, M. T. and Knorr, N. J. (1971). Motivational patterns of patients seeking cosmetic (aesthetic) surgery. *Plastic and Reconstructive Surgery*, **48**, 551–7.

Espeland, L. V. and Stenvik, A. (1991). Perception of personal dental appearance in young adults: relationship between occlusion, awareness, and satisfaction. *American Journal of Orthodontics and Dentofacial Orthopedics*, **100**, 234–41.

Esterling, B. A. (1996). Coping with cancer psychosocial problems and treatment approaches. *Journal of Practical Psychiatry and Behavioural Health*, **6**, 350–6.

Finlay, P. M., Atkinson, J. M., and Moos, K. F. (1995). Orthognathic surgery: patient expectations; psychological profile and satisfaction with outcome. *British Journal of Oral and Maxillofacial Surgery*, **33**, 9–14.

Flanary, C. M. and Alexander, J. M. (1983). Patient responses to the orthognathic surgery experience: factors leading to dissatisfaction. *Journal of Oral and Maxillofacial Surgery*, **41**, 770–4.

Flanary, C. M., Barnwell, G. M., and Alexander, J. M. (1985). Patient perceptions of orthognathic surgery. *American Journal of Orthodontics*, **88**, 137–45.

Flanary, C. M., Barnwell, G. M., Van Sickels, J. E., Littlefield, J. H., and Rugh, A. L. (1990). Impact of orthognathic surgery on normal and abnormal personality dimensions: A 2 year follow-up study of 61 patients. *American Journal of Orthodontics and Dentofacial Orthopedics*, **98**, 313–22.

Goldstein, R. A. and Lancaster, J. S. (1984). Survey of patient attitudes toward current esthetic procedures. *Journal of Prosthetic Dentistry*, **52**, 775–80.

Harper, D. C. and Richman, L. C. (1978). Personality profiles of physically impaired adolescents. *Journal of Clinical Psychology*, **34**, 636–42.

Heldt, L., Haffke, E. A., and Davis, L. F. (1982). The psychological and social aspects of orthognathic treatment. *American Journal of Orthodontics*, **82**, 318–28.

Hillerström, K., Sörenson, S., and Wictorin, L. (1971). Biological and psycho-social factors in patients with malformations of the jaws. Twelve months after maxillofacial surgery. *Scandinavian Journal of Plastic and Reconstructive Surgery*, **5**, 34–40.

Holman, A. R., Brumer, S., Ware, W. H., and Pasta, D. J. (1995). The impact of interpersonal support on patient satisfaction with orthognathic surgery. *Journal of Oral and Maxillofacial Surgery*, **53**, 1289–97.

Hutchison, I. L., Magennis, P., Shepherd, J. P., and Brown, A. E. (1998). The BAOMS United Kingdom Survey of Facial Injuries. Part I: Aetiology and the association with alcohol consumption. *British Journal of Oral and Maxillofacial Surgery*, **36**, 3–13.

Hutton, C. E. (1967). Patients' evaluation of surgical correction of prognathism: survey of 32 patients. *Journal of Oral Surgery*, **25**, 225–8.

Jacobson, A. (1984). Psychological aspects of dentofacial aesthetics and orthognathic surgery. *The Angle Orthodontist*, **54**, 18–35.

Jensen, S. H. (1978). The psychosocial dimensions of oral and maxillofacial surgery: a critical review of the literature. *Journal of Oral Surgery*, **36**, 447–53.

Kapp, K. (1979). Self concept of the cleft lip and or palate child. *Cleft Plate Journal*, **16**, 171–6.

Kapp-Simon, K. A. (1995). Psychological interventions for the adolescent with cleft lip and palate. *Cleft Palate–Craniofacial Journal*, **32**, 104–8.

Kerosuo, H., Hausen, H., Laine, T., and Shaw, W. C. (1995). The influence of incisal malocclusion on the social attractiveness of young adults in Finland. *European Journal of Orthodontics*, **17**, 505–12.

Kerr, W. J. S. and O'Donnell, J. M. (1990). Panel perception of facial attractiveness. *British Journal of Orthodontics*, **17**, 299–304.

Kiyak, H. A., Hohl, T., Sherrick, P., West, R. A., McNeill, R. W., and Bucher, F. (1981). Sex differences in motives for and outcomes of orthognathic surgery. *Journal of Oral Surgery*, **39**, 757–64.

Kiyak, H. A., McNeill, R. W., West, R. A., Hohl, T., Bucher, F., and Sherrick, P. (1982a). Predicting psychological responses to orthognathic surgery. *Journal of Oral and Maxillofacial Surgery*, **40**, 150–5.

Kiyak, H. A., West, R. A., Hohl, T., and McNeill, R. W. (1982b). The psychological impact of orthognathic surgery: a 9 month follow-up. *American Journal of Orthodontics*, **81**, 404–12.

Kiyak, H. A., Hohl, T., West, R. A., and McNeill, R. W. (1984). Psychological changes in orthognathic surgery patients: a 24 month follow-up. *Journal of Oral and Maxillofacial Surgery*, **42**, 506–12.

Kiyak, H. A., McNeill, R. W., and West, R. A. (1985). The emotional impact of orthognathic surgery and conventional orthodontics. *American Journal of Orthodontics*, **88**, 224–34.

Kiyak, H. A., McNeill, R. W., West, R. A., Hohl, T., and Heaton, P. J. (1986). Personality characteristics as predictors and sequelae of surgical and conventional orthodontics. *American Journal of Orthodontics*, **89**, 383–92.

Kurtz, R. (1969). Sex differences and variations in body attitudes. *Journal of Consulting and Clinical Psychology*, **33**, 625–9.

Lansdown, R., Lloyd, J., and Hunter, J. (1991). Facial deformity in childhood: severity and psychological adjustment. *Child: care, health and development*, **17**, 165–71.

Laufer, D., Glick, D., Gutman, D., and Sharon, A. (1976). Patient motivation and response to surgical correction of prognathism. *Oral Surgery Oral Medicine Oral Pathology*, **41**, 309–13.

Lefebvre, A. and Munro, I. (1978). The role of psychiatry in a craniofacial team. *Plastic and Reconstructive Surgery*, **61**, 546–69.

Macgregor, F. C. (1970). Social and psychological implications of dentofacial disfigurement. *The Angle Orthodontist*, **40**, 231–3.

Macgregor, F. C. (1981). Patient dissatisfaction with results of technically satisfactory surgery. *Aesthetic Plastic Surgery*, **5**, 27–32.

Magennis, P., Shepherd, J., Hutchison, I., and Brown A. (1998). Trends in facial injury. *British Medical Journal*, **316**, 325–6.

Mayou, R., Bryant, B., and Duthie, R. (1993). Psychiatric consequences of road traffic accidents. *British Medical Journal*, **307**, 647–51.

Morselli, E. (1891). Sulla dismorfofobia e sulla tafefobia. *Bolletinno della R Accademia di Genova*, **6**, 110–19.

Munjack, D. J. (1978). The behavioral treatment of dysmorphophobia. *Journal of Behavior Therapy and Experimental Psychiatry*, **9**, 53–6.

Neumann, L. M., Christensen, D., and Cavanaugh, C. (1989). Dental esthetic satisfaction in adults. *Journal of the American Dental Association*, **118**, 565–9.

Oates, A. J., Fitzgerald, M., and Alexander, G. (1995). Patient decision-making in relation to extensive restorative dental treatment. Part II: Evaluation of a patient decision-making model. *British Dental Journal*, **179**, 11–18.

Olson, M. L. and Shedd, D. P. (1978). Disability and rehabilitation in head and neck cancer patients after treatment. *Head and Neck Surgery*, **1**, 52–8.

Olson, R. E. and Laskin, D. M. (1980). Expectations of patients from orthognathic surgery. *Journal of Oral Surgery*, **38**, 283–5.

O'Regan, J. K., Dewey, M. E., Slade, P. D., and Lovius, B. B. J. (1991). Self-esteem and aesthetics. *British Journal of Orthodontics*, **18**, 111–18.

Ostler, S. and Kiyak, H. A. (1991). Treatment expectations versus outcomes among orthognathic surgery patients. *International Journal of Adult Orthodontics and Orthognathic Surgery*, **6**, 247–55.

Palkes, H. S., Marsh, J. L., and Talent, B. K. (1986). Pediatric craniofacial surgery and parental attitudes. *Cleft Plate Journal*, **23**, 137–43.

Perugi, G., Giannotti, D., Frare, F., *et al.* (1997). Prevalence, phenomenology and comorbidity of body dysmorphic disorder (dysmorphophobia) in a clinical population. *International Journal of Psychiatry in Clinical Practice*, **1**, 77–82.

Peter, J. P. and Chinsky, R. R. (1974a). Sociological aspects of cleft palate adults: I. Marriage. *Cleft Plate Journal*, **11**, 295–309.

Peter, J. P. and Chinsky, R. R. (1974b). Sociological aspects of cleft palate adults: II. Education. *Cleft Palate Journal*, **11**, 443–9.

Peter, J. P., Chinsky, R. R., and Fisher, M. J. (1975). Sociological aspects of cleft palate adults: III. Vocational and economic aspects. *Cleft Palate Journal*, **12**, 193–9.

Peterson, L. J. and Topazian, R. G. (1976). Psychological considerations in corrective maxillary and midfacial surgery. *Journal of Oral Surgery*, **34**, 157–64.

Phillips, K. A. (1991). Body dysmorphic disorder: the distress of imagined ugliness. *American Journal of Psychiatry*, **148**, 1138–49.

Phillips, K. A. and McElroy, S. L. (1993). Insight, overvalued ideation, and delusional thinking in body dysmorphic disorder: theoretical and treatment implications. *Journal of Nervous and Mental Disease*, **181**, 699–702.

Phillips, K. A., McElroy, S. L., Keck, P. E., Hudson, J. I., and Pope, H. G. (1994). A comparison of delusional and nondelusional body dysmorphic disorder in 100 cases. *Psychopharmacology Bulletin*, **30**, 179–86.

Phillips, K. A., McElroy, S. L., Hudson, J. I., and Pope, H. G. (1995). Body dysmorphic disorder: an obsessive–compulsive spectrum disorder, a form of affective spectrum disorder, or both? *Journal of Clinical Psychiatry*, **56**, (Suppl. 4), 41–51.

Prahl-Andersen, B., Boersma, H., van der Linden, F. P. G. M., and Moore, A. W. (1979). Perceptions of dentofacial morphology by laypersons, general dentists and orthodontists. *Journal of the American Dental Association*, **98**, 209–12.

Reich, J. (1969). The surgery of appearance: psychological and related aspects. *Medical Journal of Australia*, **2**, 5–8.

Reich, J. (1975). Factors influencing patient satisfaction with the results of aesthetic plastic surgery. *Plastic and Reconstructive Surgery*, **55**, 5–13.

Richman, L. C. (1983). Self-reported social, speech and facial concerns and personality adjustment of adolescents with cleft lip and palate. *Cleft Palate Journal*, **20**, 108–12.

Rittersma, J. (1989). Patient information and patient preparation in orthognathic surgery—the role of an information brochure. A medical audit study. *Journal of Craniomaxillofacial Surgery*, **17**, 278–9.

Rosen, J. C., Reiter, J., and Orosan, P. (1995). Cognitive–behavioral body image therapy for body dysmorphic disorder. *Journal of Consulting and Clinical Psychology*, **63**, 263–9.

Rumsey, N., Bull, R., and Gahagan, D. (1982). The effect of facial disfigurement on the proxemic behaviour of the general public. *Journal of Applied Social Psychology*, **12**, 137–50.

Shapiro, P. A. and Kornfeld, D. S. (1987). Psychiatric aspects of head and neck cancer surgery. *Psychiatric Clinics of North America*, **10**, 87–100.

Shaw, W. C. (1981). The influence of children's dentofacial appearance on their social attractiveness as judged by peers and lay adults. *American Journal of Orthodontics*, **79**, 399–415.

Shaw, W. C., Meek, S. C., and Jones, D. S. (1980). Nicknames, teasing, harassment and the salience of dental features among school children. *British Journal of Orthodontics*, **7**, 75–80.

Shepherd, J. P., Shapland, M., Pearce, N., and Scully, C. (1990). Pattern, severity and aetiology of injuries in assault. *Journal of the Royal Society of Medicine*, **83**, 75–8.

Solomon, S. D., Gerrity, E. T., and Muff, A. M. (1992). Efficacy of treatments for post-traumatic stress disorder: an empirical review. *Journal of the American Medical Association*, **268**, 633–8.

Stewart, T. D. and Sexton, J. (1987). Depression: a possible complication of orthognathic surgery. *Journal of Oral and Maxillofacial Surgery*, **45**, 847–51.

Thomas, C. S. (1984). Dysmorphophobia: a question of definition. *British Journal of Psychiatry*, **144**, 513–16.

Thomas, C. S. (1995). A study of facial dysmorphophobia. *Psychiatric Bulletin*, **19**, 736–9.

Thomas, C. S. and Goldberg, D. P. (1995). Appearance, body image and distress in facial dysmorphophobia. *Acta Psychiatrica Scandinavica*, **92**, 231–6.

Varela, M. and Garcia-Camba, J. E. (1995). Impact of orthodontics on the psychological profile of adult patients: a prospective study. *American Journal of Orthodontics and Dentofacial Orthopedics*, **108**, 142–8.

Veale, D., Boocock, A., Gournay, K., *et al.* (1996). Body dysmorphic disorder; a survey of fifty cases. *British Journal of Psychiatry*, **169**, 196–201.

West, D. W. (1977). Social adaptation patterns among cancer patients with facial disfigurements resulting from surgery. *Archives of Physical and Medical Rehabilitation*, **58**, 473–9.

Wictorin, L., Hillerström, K., and Sörenson, S. (1969). Biological and psycho-social factors in patients with malformation of the jaws: a study of 95 patients prior to treatment. *Scandinavian Journal of Plastic and Reconstructive Surgery*, **3**, 138–143.

World Health Organization (1992). *The ICD-10 Classification of mental and behavioural disorders; clinical descriptions and diagnostic guidelines*. WHO, Geneva.

Appendix 1

Fabrication of a full coverage occlusal splint

Richard Ibbetson

PRACTICAL ADVICE ON CONSTRUCTION OF AN OCCLUSAL APPLIANCE

A wide variety of appliances has been described. If the recommendations that appliances should provide a reversible form of treatment are to be followed, the choice becomes more limited. The splint should cover all of the teeth in the arch where it is fitted and should provide stable contacts on closure for all the teeth in the opposing arch. This essentially limits the choice to either a full-coverage maxillary or mandibular appliance. Each has its advocates and there are no definite contraindications to either type. It is generally true that the adjustment and monitoring of a maxillary splint is easier than for a similar mandibular appliance. However, the maxillary splint presents more bulk to the patient and is sometimes not the correct choice on this account. Provision of a well-designed maxillary occlusal splint in patients who have a significant horizontal overlap of the anterior teeth will make the anterior portion of the splint bulky and thick. The same is true for patients who have a class III incisor relationship. In both these instances, a mandibular appliance is to be preferred. A further consideration in making a choice between a maxillary or mandibular appliance is whether there are missing teeth and their location. If teeth are absent, it may be sensible to make the appliance for the arch where tooth loss has occurred as the splint can replace these in a temporary way: this will assist in achieving the occlusal requirements for the appliance. Whether it be mandibular or maxillary, it should fulfil the criteria for an ideal occlusion for the natural dentition and provide:

- stable contacts on mandibular closure;
- sufficient anterior guidance to separate the posterior teeth on mandibular movement.

Such an appliance when constructed for the maxillary arch will provide a relatively even and generally flat surface posteriorly. The surface will be free of indentations so that the mandible is not constrained into a particular position on closure. There will usually be a gentle ramp just on the front portion of the splint. On mandibular movement, the gentle curvature of this ramp will allow the anterior teeth to assist in separating the posterior teeth from their contact with the splint. The anterior guidance and the form of the splint posteriorly will ensure that the posterior teeth do not contact the appliance in any excursive position of the mandible. The acrylic resin should lip over the incisal edges of the maxillary anterior teeth by approximately 1 mm, to ensure that the appliance cannot act like a functional orthodontic appliance to push the upper anterior teeth labially. Posteriorly the acrylic resin can be terminated level with the buccal cusp tips. It may, however, be extended a little onto the buccal surfaces of the posterior teeth: this makes the appliance more retentive but can also sometimes make it more difficult to seat.

The extension of the acrylic resin onto the buccal surfaces of the posterior teeth is indicated when the clinical crowns are relatively short and, consequently, retention might be in short supply. These appliances do not need retentive devices, such as clasps or Adam's cribs, to be incorporated into their design: the splint makes use of the natural undercuts on the teeth for its retention. The appliance is best constructed using heat-cured acrylic resin to provide a hard, durable surface and an appliance with low levels of residual acrylic monomer.

If the appliance is made for the mandibular arch, the design principles will be the same. However, the anterior ramp of acrylic resin will cover part of the incisal edges and facial surfaces of the lower anterior teeth to provide the disclusion of the posterior teeth on mandibular movement. The position of the anterior ramp can give difficulties in adjusting the anterior guidance on the appliance as the position of the acrylic resin makes it more difficult to keep the anterior guidance shallow. A further concern has been expressed that the additional bulk of acrylic resin covering the mandibular anterior teeth can act to move the maxillary anterior teeth labially. However, there are no records of this theoretical risk becoming a practical reality.

Each type of appliance requires that an accurate set of study casts is made and that the maxillary cast should be mounted in a semi-adjustable articulator using a facebow transfer. Casts made from accurate alginate impressions will suffice as long as the impressions are made and poured with care. An impression tray must be selected which is rigid, and therefore generally made of metal. It must also cover the surfaces of all the teeth in one arch. It is frequently observed that the most distal tooth in the arch is recorded by impression material which extends beyond the posterior border of the tray. Such alginate is unsupported and will be distorted by placing the impression face-up on a work surface or by pouring stone into it. It is best practice to use a sharp scalpel after the impression is removed from the mouth to remove all impression material which extends beyond the border of the tray. Hence the need to use a tray that has sufficient extension to cover all the teeth in the arch.

Surface detail of the alginate impression is improved by ensuring that the teeth are dry before the impression is made. This is most easily achieved by wiping the teeth thoroughly with an absorbent tissue as the alginate material is being mixed. It is also helpful, while the dental nurse is loading the impression tray, to use a finger to wipe the alginate into the functional surfaces of the teeth. A regular-setting alginate is required: fast-setting materials will cause the material wiped directly onto the teeth to be partially set when the tray is seated.

On separating the impression from the teeth, a check should be made to ensure that the material has not become partially detached from the tray. If it has, the impression should be discarded and remade. A further check should be made to see that a tooth has not contacted the internal surface of the tray. If it has, the impression should again be remade, as pouring the impression will result in stone percolating between the tray and impression material, distorting the cast.

RELATING THE CASTS

The maxillary casts are mounted in a semi-adjustable articulator using a facebow transfer. The mandibular cast should be mounted against the maxillary cast using an interocclusal record, made with an anterior jig in place to record as accurately as possible the retruded axis position. However, in patients suffering from temporomandibular dysfunction, manipulation of the mandible into a true retruded axis position is likely to be difficult, inaccurate, and can sometimes be very uncomfortable for the patient. It is reasonable, under these circumstances, to consider relating the casts in the articulator in the intercuspal position. However, this is done in the knowledge that increased adjustment of the occlusal splint will be necessary on fitting the appliance and possibly also at the initial review appointments.

The occlusal splint is waxed by the technician. The casts must be separated sufficiently to allow the splint to be of approximately 1 mm thickness over the last molars. There will otherwise generally not be sufficient acrylic resin thickness to make it durable. The splint is then invested and processed before the cast is returned to the articulator for any necessary adjustment prior to polishing.

FITTING THE SPLINT

The dentist should examine the splint carefully before fitting. In particular, any nodules of acrylic resin on the fitting surface of the appliance should be removed. These may not only impede seating but may risk fracturing a tooth if they act on a weakened cusp. The splint may feel tight on the teeth at first: the patient should be encouraged to bear with this aspect as following a short period of wear it will become looser. If the splint does not seat, it may be that an undercut on one or more of the teeth is responsible. Careful adjustment of the acrylic resin in apposition to the mesio-palatal aspects of the posterior teeth may relieve these. Failure to seat may also be due to a distortion of the impression: if attempts to adjust the internal aspect of the splint do not prove successful, a remake of the splint is probably necessary. The patient should not be provided with an occlusal splint that is anything other than stable on closure and mandibular movement.

The splint will generally require adjustment to ensure that the criteria for the occlusal scheme are met. In adjusting the splint, indentations at the sites of occlusal contact should not be created. These will tend to reinforce a particular position of closure on the mandible which will hinder successful use of the appliance. It is generally wise to adjust the splint in the retruded axis position first: the aim being to ensure that each posterior tooth has a minimum of one contact with the splint. Sometimes teeth will be encountered that are well below the level of the occlusal plane: occasionally it may be reasonable to leave a solitary tooth in this position out of contact, but there remains the risk of unwanted axial tooth movement. The excursive movements are then adjusted: the aim is to provide gentle anterior guidance which is sufficient to separate the posterior teeth when the mandible moves. The most common error is to make the anterior guidance too steep initially, the first part of the movement controlled by the splint should be shallow.

In general, the partial-coverage appliances, including the mandibular repositioning appliances and posterior bite planes, are not recommended, due to potential tooth movement (Ramfjord and Ash 1995). The stabilization appliances essentially provide reversible therapy with no permanent occlusal changes. Further investigation with well-controlled randomized clinical trials are still required in this field.

REFERENCE

Ramfjord, S. P. and Ash, M. M. Jr (1995). *Occlusion*, (4th edn). W. B. Saunders, Philadelphia.

Appendix 2

Information on facial pain

Charlotte Feinmann

This information leaflet has been designed to help you to understand your problem.
Toothache and other dental problems are fairly straightforward to explain.
They respond to simple treatments and do not recur.
Other pains may develop as a reaction to stress or without any obvious cause.

FACIAL ARTHROMYALGIA (TEMPOROMANDIBULAR JOINT DYSFUNCTION SYNDROME)

This is a dull ache with occasional severe attacks affecting the jaw joint and its muscles.
You may also experience other symptoms, such as clicking in the joint, difficulty opening the mouth, and spasm in the jaw muscles which extend into the head and down into the neck.
Ear symptoms such as a sense of fullness or buzzing and dizziness are also possible.

ATYPICAL FACIAL PAIN (IDIOPATHIC FACIAL PAIN)

This is a dull ache or sharp pain, affecting the cheeks, eyes, jaws and all non-muscular parts of the face.
The pain may come and go and may be worse when you are tired and under stress.

ATYPICAL ODONTALGIA

This is a pain or severe discomfort in the teeth or in the tooth socket after an extraction, in the absence of any usual dental cause.

The pain may be made worse by dental treatment and can move from tooth to tooth.

ORAL DYSAESTHESIA

This is a group of problems that include a burning or altered sensation in the tongue or gums or a nasty taste. You may notice a sense of increased or decreased saliva in the mouth. It may be difficult for you to wear dentures or tolerate new fillings, crowns, or bridges, despite many attempts to help you.

PHANTOM BITE SYNDROME

This is an unpleasant awareness that your teeth do not meet comfortably. This does not respond to balancing the occlusion.

These problems often last for long periods of time and will come and go when you are under stress. The situations that particularly affect us are long-term problems, such as difficulties with our children, our work, housing, marital strain, being lonely, ill health in the family, or more upsetting events such as bereavement, divorce, or moving house. It may surprise you to know, that getting married, being promoted, or having a baby are also events that put us under stress.

Children may develop such pains as a result of marital dysharmony or poor adaptation to school.

Many patients also find that they suffer from other stress-related problems, such as tension headaches and neckache, migraine, chronic low back pain, pelvic pain or painful periods, stomach pains (especially irritable bowel), and itchy skin. All of these problems suggest that emotional stress causes widespread symptoms in certain susceptible individuals.

TREATMENT

In order to make a diagnosis, we need to take a full, detailed history and sometimes do blood tests and X-rays. It is important that you understand that the diagnosis of these pains does not mean that we think you are imagining your pain.

The pain is real and arises in cramped muscles and dilated blood vessels.

We prescribe antidepressant drugs for these pains **NOT** because we think you are depressed **but because we have shown that this medication helps to prevent the pain.**

You will need to take medication for some months to ensure relief. It is **NOT** addictive and has no serious side-effects, although, depending on the medication prescribed, some patients may initially experience drowsiness, dry mouth, or occasional constipation.

If you have any questions, please ask us or your doctor.

Professor Malcolm Harris   Dr Charlotte Feinmann

Appendix 3

Management of facial pain problems by the practitioner

Charlotte Feinmann

Your patient has been told that he/she has a stress-related pain in the face.
Although most dental problems are fairly straightforward to diagnose and respond to simple therapy, idiopathic pains or those that develop as a reaction to stress are more complicated to diagnose and treat.
The diagnosis of idiopathic facial pain is based on the following presentations:

FACIAL ARTHROMYALGIA (TEMPOROMANDIBULAR JOINT DYSFUNCTION SYNDROME; COSTEN'S SYNDROME)

This is a dull ache with occasional severe attacks affecting the jaw joint and its muscles. The patient may also experience other symptoms, such as clicking and sticking in the joint, trismus, and pain in the jaw muscles which extends into the head and down into the neck. Ear symptoms such as a sense of fullness, or buzzing and dizziness, are also possible.

IDIOPATHIC FACIAL PAIN (ATYPICAL FACIAL PAIN)

This is a dull ache or sharp pain affecting the cheeks, eyes, jaws, and non-muscular parts of the face. The pain is intermittent and may be worse when the patient is tired and under stress. The pain can be unilateral or bilateral and persists for many months or years. There are no detectable neurological signs.

ATYPICAL ODONTALGIA

This is a pain in the teeth or in the tooth socket, in the absence of any usual dental cause. It may be made worse by dental treatment and can move from tooth to tooth. When the teeth are extracted the pain persists as an atypical facial pain.

ORAL DYSAESTHESIA

This group includes a burning or altered sensation in the tongue (glossodynia or glossopyrosis), gums, or lips, or a nasty taste. Some patients have a sense of increased or decreased salivation. It may also be difficult for the patient to wear dentures or tolerate new restorations, crowns, or bridges, despite many attempts to help.

PHANTOM BITE SYNDROME

Another related problem is the phantom bite syndrome—an unpleasant awareness that the teeth do not meet comfortably. This persists despite many attempts to balance the occlusion.

These pains persist for long periods of time and will come and go when the patient is under stress. The situations that can be related to the onset of symptoms in children are parental marital dysharmony or poor adaptation to school. In adults, precipitating situations include social isolation, housing, occupational and marital problems, or chronic ill health in the family, or more acute upsetting events such as bereavement, divorce, or moving house.

Getting married, being promoted, or having a baby are also events that may precipitate orofacial pain.

Many patients also suffer from related problems such as tension headaches, neckache, chronic low back pain, dysmenorrhoea, irritable bowel, pelvic pain, and pruritis. All suggest that emotional stress causes widespread symptoms in certain susceptible individuals.

MANAGEMENT AND TREATMENT

Our investigations have excluded a structural problem but it is important to emphasize that the diagnosis does not imply an imaginary pain. The pain is real and is described as arising in cramped muscles and dilated blood vessels as a response to stress.

Antidepressant drugs relieve these pains independently of any effect on depression, which is not always present. The patient may need medication for six or more months to ensure relief. It is our experience that the drugs are not addictive and have no serious side-effects, although some may suffer drowsiness, a dry mouth, or occasionally constipation.

A CONSENSUS THERAPEUTIC APPROACH

1.   Informed reassurance, occasional analgesia (NSAIDs) or paracetamol are usually sufficient in 50 per cent of patients.

2.   Tricyclic antidepressants should be prescribed at night, in slowly increasing doses, combined with regular review at 3–6-week intervals to provide reassurance and achieve compliance. As sedation is not required in most cases, a drug with low sedative and low anticholinergic side-effects, such as nortriptyline, is recommended. Nortriptyline may be increased gradually from 10 to 100 mg.

   (a) With insomnia, the more sedative drug dothiepin may be given at night (25 mg, increased to 225 mg when necessary).

   (b) In elderly patients with constipation and glaucoma, and in males with prostatic hypertrophy, the least anticholinergic drug should be prescribed. The selective serotonin reuptake inhibitors, such as fluoxetine 20–60 mg mane, offer a suitable alternative.

   (c) A combination of drugs such as nortriptyline and a phenothiazine is useful when the patients pain is accompanied by extreme anxiety or bizarre symptoms. Trifluoperazine (2 mg three times a day) or flupenthixol or fluphenazine (0.5–1.5 mg twice a day) may be used and increased as the symptoms dictate.

   (d) When there is no response to tricyclics, MAOIs are sometimes employed, e.g. tranylcypromine 10–20 mg twice a day.

3.   Arthroscopy is indicated in cases of persistent limitation of opening and internal derangement of the joint.

4.   Patients with complex emotional histories, depression, agitated, or psychotic states are referred to our liaison psychiatrist.

5.   For intractable pain we recommend cognitive therapy with or without medication.

SUMMARY

Stoicism is often required on the part of the clinician, as those patients for whom medication is essential are often resistant to this management and complain of more side-effects. Pain recurrence is often associated with withdrawal of medication, and in some cases medication has to be continued to prevent relapse. Once the patient has confidence in the medication and has been free from pain for 23 months, it can usually be reduced without problems.

Idiopathic facial pain should be considered to be a chronic disturbance, such as trigeminal neuralgia or migraine, and be treated when necessary with a comparable, continuous medical regime.

Professor Malcolm Harris   Dr Charlotte Feinmann

Index